Paradox and Imperatives in Health Care

How Efficiency, Effectiveness, and E-Transformation Can Conquer Waste and Optimize Quality

Jeffrey C. Bauer, PhD
Mark Hagland

Foreword by David B. Nash, MD, MBA

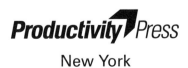

Productivity Press

New York

Most Productivity Press books are available at quantity discounts when purchased in bulk. For more information contact our Customer Service Department (888-319-5852). Address all other inquiries to:

Productivity Press
444 Park Avenue South, 7th Floor
New York, NY 10016
United States of America
Telephone: 212-686-5900
Fax: 212-686-5411
E-mail: info@productivitypress.com
ProductivityPress.com

Library of Congress Cataloging-in-Publication Data

Bauer, Jeffrey C.
    Paradox and imperatives in health care : how efficiency, effectiveness, and e-transformation can conquer waste and optimize quality / by Jeffrey C. Bauer, Mark Hagland ; foreword by David B. Nash.
        p. ; cm.
    Includes index.
    ISBN 978-1-56327-379-7 (alk. paper)
    1. Health services administration—Economic aspects. 2. Organizational effectiveness. 3. Organizational change. 4. Health care reform. 5. Medical care—Cost effectiveness. 6. Medical care—Quality control. I. Hagland, Mark. II. Title.
    [DNLM: 1. Efficiency, Organizational. 2. Hospital Administration—economics. 3. Health Care Reform. 4. Information Management. 5. Organizational Innovation--economics. WX 157 B3435p 2008]
    RA971.3.B377 2008
    362.1068—dc22

                                                          2007039182

12   11   10   09   08   5   4   3   2   1

This book is dedicated to
Elizabeth Bauer and to John von Rhein

CONTENTS

FOREWORD

Jeff Bauer and Mark Hagland had me at hello! Having known them both for more than 15 years, I had a good feeling that their new book would be a veritable treasure trove of important pearls of wisdom for senior health care leaders across the system. They have not disappointed me. *Paradox and Imperatives in Health Care* is going to be a watershed read for many individuals. It takes aspects of the prevailing wisdom in our industry and deconstructs it with solid economic thinking and a taut analysis akin to a graduate seminar in a leading business school. Bauer and Hagland are at once complementary with their skill sets and unlikely bedfellows: the scholar and the journalist working together to really get to the bottom of things, eliminate the jargon, and tell us what we really need to know.

The core of the book is its collective call for a major shift in thinking for provider organizations like mine, Thomas Jefferson University and Thomas Jefferson University Hospital (Jefferson Health System), in Philadelphia. The authors challenge us to perform as well as possible with inconsistent and uncontrolled work processes (effectiveness with quality as a variable) and to deliver exactly what is promised with standardized work processes (effectiveness with quality as a fixed constraint). They wisely recognize that the strategic implications of their conclusion represent a radical challenge to the *status quo*. Machiavelli knew, five centuries ago, that those who challenge the status quo have a great deal to lose.

For example, the follow-on from their aforementioned conclusion is that pay for performance (P4P) thresholds are not much of a stretch from our traditional baseline, and that reimbursement reform will not work either. What are we to do then? Here, Bauer and Hagland claim that providers need to intervene directly in the production of medical services and, they need to accomplish this clinical transformation on their own sooner, rather than later, because "meaningful industry-wide solutions are unlikely to occur in the current political and economic environment."

So, we need a radical change in the status quo, and P4P in reimbursement reform will not work. What will? Here is where I really appreciate this collective work, because the authors unabashedly have selected quality as the fundamental criterion to measure effectiveness in the American health care delivery system. They view quality in an interesting, novel, and compelling way—as the centerpiece of a response to their effectiveness imperative. In other words, quantifying quality has become their mantra. They rightly indicate that our decades-old reliance on structure and process measures simply will not prove adequate for the future. They call for hospitals and medical groups to produce honest numbers to support prespecified claims of providing quality. Without this supportive data, the typical mission statements about quality will be meaningless.

Now comes the hard part. By casting quality in terms of effectiveness, efficiency, and the elimination of waste, they have set a high bar for performance moving forward. Here is where Hagland's interviews with successful leaders and their systems around the country come into play. By cleverly weaving the economic analysis together with tantalizing examples of how to meet the challenges, the authors have strung together a group of clinical and economic pearls to make, if you would, a beautiful necklace.

I think most system leaders, after finishing this book, will ask themselves four difficult questions consistent with the four levels of analysis that Bauer and Hagland weave throughout the text. The first question might go something like: "Are we able to identify and reallocate all the wasted resources in our delivery system?" The second question, just as tough, might be something like: "Can we capture the opportunity costs of the disorganized production process?" Health care leaders will find it hard, in my view, to redirect resources to produce less expensive and top-quality services. The third question might read: "Of all the lists of impending e-technologies like electronic medical records, which ones provide the most return on our investment?" Mounting evidence is checkered regarding how we might calculate, in current terms, the greatest return in this sphere. The fourth and final question is probably the toughest: "Do we have the right organizational structure in place to respond to the imperatives of the future medical marketplace?" Here is where Bauer and Hagland really put stress on the status quo, as trustees and senior executives will be forced to oversee the transformation from fighting external threats to guiding internal changes that lower costs and improve outcomes. It is so much easier to blame an outside force than it is to conduct the real business we are in.

Hats off to Bauer and Hagland for a tough job well done! I am confident that this book will have the power to change the current conversation about health care and apply a rigorous economic framework to our fuzzy current thinking. I am equally confident that many leaders will become naysayers after having read this book steadfast in their defense of the status quo. I am convinced that our status quo is untenable, and I am hopeful that Bauer and Hagland will be widely read and more importantly, heard.

Readers will do what I did when I had the privilege of reviewing the final draft. They will scratch their heads, talk out loud, phone a friend, and by the last page, scribble notes in the margin regarding what they might do differently come Monday morning. I am hopeful that all those collective scribbles will create a *chain* of pearl necklaces, tightly woven, able to withstand great pressures, and to collectively lead us, successfully, into the remainder of the 21st century.

David B. Nash, MD, MBA, FACP
The Raymond C. & Doris N. Grandon Professor & Chair,
Department of Health Policy, Jefferson Medical College,
Thomas Jefferson University
Philadelphia, Pennsylvania

PREFACE

*Surely we will end up where we are headed
if we do not change direction.*

—*Confucius*

When we decided to write a book about health care's high costs and inconsistent quality and what should be done to stop this embarrassing waste, we asked a diverse sample of industry leaders for their reactions. Several executives responded with a question: "Why would a provider want to cut costs or improve quality?" After all, they argued, the reimbursement system doesn't provide incentives to reduce costs, and the rewards for quality can be relatively small with respect to the required effort. Reimbursement can even penalize performance improvement initiatives. They indicated no interest in reading a book on efficiency and effectiveness until the federal government required them to take action.

Several executives took an opposite position. They believed our proposed focus was important—so important that they had, in their opinions, already removed all the waste from their organizations. They probably would not read our book because there was nothing more they could do to save money in operations. Nevertheless, without seeing that there's *always* room for improvement, they encouraged us to write it because they thought other hospitals needed the message.

Ultimately, we wrote the book because most executives were in the middle, skeptical but receptive to new perspectives and responsive solutions. They acknowledged the disincentives that have thwarted past efforts to change a production process or business model. They also sensed an unprecedented convergence of forces that compelled action. They wanted a practical guide that would help them survive and, hopefully, thrive in a potentially hostile marketplace.

The Threat

Dark clouds commonly hover over the medical marketplace, but they have had a silver lining in the past. Intense political action could always reverse announced cuts in government programs. Playing hardball with managed care plans would ultimately yield a viable contract. Better collections procedures could manage receivables and cash flow. Keeping revenue above expenses was never easy, but with hard work in the finance department, it could be accomplished.

Something in this equation has changed over the past year or two. Tighter government reimbursement and rapid increases in consumers' financial responsibility started creating an uncommonly gloomy outlook for revenue. High-deductible health insurance plans have suddenly become the norm. Receivables have begun rising precipitously, even for patients covered by the better commercial health plans. Costs for supplies and labor are increasing, too. Regulations never cease to grow in number and complexity. Troubling trends in the national and international economies cast doubt on any prospects for improvement in public or private capacity to pay for health care. And medical tourism is suddenly drawing a noticeable number of reliable self-pay patients to hospitals in other countries.

The Imperative

Hospitals, medical groups, and integrated health systems rightly feel under siege. The external dangers are real and present. However, no mounted cavalry is approaching to save health care from this assault. The purchasers (government and business) who rode to the rescue in the past don't have any spare resources to help now or in the foreseeable future. The underlying circumstances are different this time. Learning to "game the system" or complaining about the obvious injustices of reimbursement won't work any more. Instead, providers must start drawing upon their own resources and resourcefulness to survive.

Fortunately, providers have an internal resource to draw upon—the pervasive waste generated by inefficient and ineffective production processes on the supply side of the medical marketplace. Resources are abundantly, even shamelessly, wasted in the production of health care services. The transformative process of redirecting wasted resources to productive use within the enterprise is the central focus of this book. Becoming efficient and effective is the only way that the vast majority of providers will stay in business, as payers reach the limits of what they are willing and able to pay.

The reimbursement system is also wasteful, but history and politics suggest quite convincingly that third-party payment will not be reformed any time soon. Providers that place their bets on external payment reform rather than internal economic transformation will be lucky to survive in the new, emerging medical marketplace. Payers do not readily admit their indisputable contribution to the high costs of health care, but they have the power of the purse. Their attacks on providers' high costs and inconsistent quality will set the stage for the next act in the drama of health care, reinforcing the imperative for providers to play their roles efficiently and effectively—or get off the stage.

Analytical Foundation for Solutions

This book integrates four levels of analysis that collectively explain why and how health care organizations must transform their internal operations to survive in the new marketplace.

The first level of analysis explains why providers must identify and reallocate wasted resources as an essential precondition of economic survival. It methodically identifies political and economic realities that will not welcome "business as usual" (i.e., wasteful production processes) in hospitals and medical groups. Evaluation of key trends, both internal and external, shows that the future will differ significantly from the past. Providers must develop new responses to new circumstances because strategies that worked in the past are increasingly irrelevant. The myth of imminent payment reform is laid to rest, allowing organizational leadership to focus on the forces it can control.

The second level of analysis delves directly into the issues around the waste that exists throughout the health care delivery system. Economic concepts of efficiency and effectiveness are applied in practical terms to expose the remarkable volume of resources that could be redirected to produce less expensive and top-quality health care services. This analysis regularly addresses the opportunity costs of disorganized production processes—that is, the better economic and clinical results that could be achieved if wasted resources were redirected to productive use.

The third analytical level explores and explains proven processes for efficient and effective production, including appropriate adoption of e-technologies (e.g., electronic medical records, bar-coding for drug administration, charge capture, and remote presence systems). It applies important lessons that can be learned from other industries forced to change in order to stay in business when customers were no longer willing to deal on traditional terms. Numerous case studies are used to show how pioneering health care delivery organizations are reaping the benefits of performance improvement tools, including lean management and Six Sigma.

The fourth level of analysis explores leadership's strategic role in structuring organizational responses to the new imperatives of the medical marketplace. It shows how trustees and senior executives can initiate and oversee the necessary transformation, from fighting external threats to guiding internal changes that lower costs and improve outcomes—the real business of health care.

These levels of analysis are interwoven throughout the book. Each chapter incorporates some concepts from all four perspectives. The final chapter presents an integrated summary in the form of a call to action. Our book's ultimate goal is to put the health care delivery system on a positive path, while redirection is still attainable, because the current course is headed in a negative direction.

The Target Audience

This book is written primarily for the leaders of hospitals, medical groups, and health systems. The content is specifically presented from a strategic perspective, giving decision makers enough knowledge to recognize changes that must be considered and can be made. Board members, senior executives, and chief clinical officers will find the information they need to set a new course, to hire content experts to manage the journey, and to hold these experts accountable for the success of the work. In other words, this book prepares leaders for decisions about what needs to be done and offers tools to operate efficiently and effectively. It is not an in-depth guide for managing the daily tasks of performance improvement. For leaders who have the time and desire to learn more about the tactics of performance improvement, the book includes references to appropriate publications and organizations.

Although the target audience is health care's decision makers, this book should be equally valuable to employers, policy analysts, purchasers, patients, and other stakeholders who have a direct interest in ensuring quality in the medical marketplace. It can be used as a resource for improving the strained relations between customers on the demand side and providers on the supply side. Hospitals and medical groups will regain consumers' respect by improving the way they do business—putting these institutions in a position to demand adequate reimbursement once they can prove they are operating efficiently and effectively. Visionary leaders on the demand side of the market should use this book to start imagining how all stakeholders could collaborate to create exemplary health care in the United States.

The Authors' Roles

We two authors, Jeff Bauer and Mark Hagland, bring different and complementary backgrounds to this book. Bauer has spent half his 35-year career in health care as a professor of economics, statistics, and research at two academic medical centers. He has worked for national consulting firms for the other half of his career, predominantly as a health futurist and industry thought leader. He is widely recognized for his creative, "big picture" insights into evolution of the delivery system. Hagland has been a full-time, national award-winning health care journalist for nearly 20 years. He is a prolific chronicler of the day-to-day story of health care, having contributed more than 1,500 articles to the industry's major trade publications on a wide range of topics. Every week, he interviews leading health care professionals and reports on and analyzes their activities for thousands of readers.

We combined our different skills as scholar and journalist to write a more comprehensive work than anything either of us could have written alone. The primary authorship of many sections will be evident by the focus on theory and strategy (Bauer) or practice and results (Hagland). However, we have jointly authored several chapters of this book with ease because we had reached the same conclusions before deciding to write a book together.

We share serious concerns about the mounting threats to providers…and optimistic expectations that the majority will overcome them by reallocating wasted resources to productive use. We would not have taken on this gargantuan task if we did not believe that the book's prescriptions could help progressive providers survive the tough times immediately ahead and thrive in the long run. We have enormous respect for the pragmatic and innovative leaders responsible for the future of our hospitals and medical groups. We wrote this book as our contribution to the success of these individuals in preserving a critical sector of the American economy.

ACKNOWLEDGMENTS

We gratefully acknowledge (Bauer's) colleagues at ACS-Healthcare Solutions who shared their valuable experience in performance improvement, management engineering, and clinical transformation: Charles Bracken, Todd Wright, Arvind Kumar, Steve Gray, Seth Sharpe, Paul Solverson, Dr. B. J. Bomentre, Laura Dorenfest, Toni DiVizio, and Anthony Manino. We also thank the clinician leaders, executives, managers, and communications professionals at the following organizations for their exceptional cooperation with our research and reporting for this book: Brigham & Women's Hospital, Boston; Virginia Commonwealth University Health System, Richmond; Allegheny General Hospital, Pittsburgh; Virginia Mason Medical Center, Seattle; Genesys Health System, Flint, Michigan; Crystal Run Health Care, Middletown, New York; Geisinger Health System, Danville, Pennsylvania; New York-Presbyterian Hospital, New York, New York; Fairview Health Services, Minneapolis; Hackensack (New Jersey) Medical Center; Memorial Sloan-Kettering Cancer Center, New York, New York; and Hill Physicians Medical Group, San Ramon, California. Finally, we thank generous colleagues at Toyota Motor Manufacturing Kentucky, Inc.; Jeffrey K. Liker, PhD, of the University of Michigan, Ann Arbor, Michigan; Brian Parrish at Dodge Communications; Angela Lipscomb of SAS; and outside reviewers Dr. William T. Brown, Dr. Margaret Schulte, Dr. Allen Goldberg, Dr. Hunt Kooiker, Lois Huminiak, and Frank Bauer.

| ONE |

THE ECONOMIC CHALLENGE: APPROACHING CHAOS

The opening line from a famous Charles Dickens novel has been popular in recent commentaries on health care. The paradox of "the best of times" and "the worst of times" undoubtedly resonates with the trustees and executives of most health care delivery organizations. Belts are tight, but nobody is starving. A few persistent financial problems have even been brought under control; further, some serious threats have not materialized as had been predicted just a few years ago. Times could be a little better for hospitals and medical groups, but they could also be a lot worse. Providers seem to be generally comfortable with their current strategies. Few are voluntarily undertaking drastic actions to prepare for rough times ahead.

Although the balance between good and bad may be generally acceptable for now, the economic infrastructure that supports the medical marketplace is exhibiting some ominous signs. The majority of providers may need to think of today's mixed signals as the calm before a storm—an approaching Class 5 storm with the potential to demolish unprepared organizations. This time, the signals are not a false alarm. They indicate fundamental economic changes that will likely create unprecedented outcomes. These new outcomes call for unprecedented responses, sooner rather than later.

Leaders need to prepare for the possibility that health care's historic ability to survive external threats by holding firm (i.e., simply maintaining the status quo) has ended. Purchasers, payers, and policy-makers could always afford to compromise after challenging the provider community in the past. Their own economic growth allowed them to spend a little more on health care once the dust settled, even after they said they would not. Reform-minded payers who threatened permanent cuts in reimbursement were taken as seriously as the boy who cried wolf. Besides, the bark was always worse than the bite.

All parties in the medical marketplace survived with a constant portion when the "pie" was growing, but many indicators suggest that the size of the pie is not going to get any larger in the foreseeable future. The positive news is that the pie is not expected to shrink. However, the era has ended where providers could count on getting small increases after threats of big reductions. The groups paying the bills have reached their limits for a variety of economic reasons. Providers need to prepare for this equivalent of a major climatic event: the end of rising incomes. This book is a guide for weathering the storm.

Situation Not Hopeless, but Response Required

To avoid losing readers who avoid bad news, we reflect on Parson Malthus' characterization of economics as "the dismal science." (Dismal because unchecked natural forces inevitably lead to famine and misery.) Fortunately, the science of economics subsequently developed to pursue better outcomes. Good economists use theory to prescribe good practices. *Even if our forecast of a perfect economic storm turns out to be wrong, the preparations we recommend will be appropriate under any circumstances.*

Hospitals and medical groups should take the recommended steps to become efficient and effective even if no economic threats lie on the horizon. The waste in health care—measured in high cost and low quality—is becoming unacceptable to the people who pay the bills. They believe the causes of inefficient and ineffective health care should be swept away, which is one major reason why an economic storm is brewing. If providers, with power to improve health care from within, refuse to make the necessary changes, then outsiders will impose other solutions that would be better described as recurring nightmares rather than passing storms.

Most providers likely have a few years to get their economic act in order. Hence, the "take-home" point is not so much the warning that an approaching economic storm will ravage unprepared providers, but that those who prepare for it appropriately will create a much better delivery system. Denial and inaction mask an opportunity to produce better health care and healthier Americans by reallocating wasted resources to productive use. The opportunity to implement real solutions to serious problems is exciting. Professional pride alone should spur health care's leaders into action.

Not a Prediction

This book's focus on a serious economic disturbance—the end of buyers' willingness and ability to keep paying more for health care, as in the past, and the resulting end of revenue growth for providers—is a forecast, not a prediction. Predictions and forecasts are decidedly not the same thing. The difference between them merits a quick explanation because predictions are becoming meaningless in today's medical marketplace. Unfortunately, most comments about the future of health care are made as predictions.

A prediction states what will happen at a specific time in the future, such as: health care spending will reach 20 percent of the gross domestic product in 2015. Predictions are mathematical extrapolations made from historical data. An equation determines the "best fit" for the relationship between the variables in the past and computes future values based on the assumption that the past relationship will continue. Many readers will remember using linear regression analysis to make predictions when they took quantitative analysis courses in graduate school (often, an unpleasant memory). The accuracy of predictions depends completely on the assumption that the historical relationship will continue. Changes in the explanatory relationships weaken the predictive value of the equation. The more these relationships change, the less meaningful the prediction becomes.

Well, the key explanatory relationships in health care are now changing at an accelerating rate. For example, the one-size-fits-all, symptom-based medical care of the 20th century is being replaced by personalized, biology-based diagnostics and treatments. The demographic, cultural, and racial diversification of the U.S. population is changing the types of diseases that providers treat. Demand is also redirected by the shift of significant financial responsibility from payers to consumers. The growing number of nontraditional sites of care, like investor-owned surgery centers and retail-based primary care clinics staffed by nurse practitioners, now draws income away from traditional providers.

None of these new forces is reflected in the historical data on which predictions are based. The predictions become correspondingly meaningless because the consistency assumption behind predictive models is violated. The principal assumption behind this book, the stabilization of providers' real incomes, is sufficient reason to discard predicting as a way to assess its impact. Another approach is needed.

Forecasting Is the Tool to Use

Leaders need a different tool when key relationships move in unexpected directions. Fortunately, sciences that deal with change and uncertainty, such as physics and meteorology, have perfected forecasting as an alternative to predicting. Forecasting is ideal for looking at the future of health care because the medical economy is changing fast and, literally, unpredictably. However, forecasting is almost never included in training programs for health care executives. Teaching how to make predictions was considered appropriate when health care was changing relatively little over the last half of the 20th century. A quick overview of forecasting is important, now that all the key relationships are changing rapidly. Executives and trustees need to know just enough to call upon experts to help them forecast, not predict, the future.

Forecasts are estimates of the probabilities of possibilities. In direct contrast to predictions that posit one outcome at a specific time in the future, forecasts assign probabilities to each of the possible outcomes. In other words, forecasts present the likelihood of different future scenarios, which clearly makes them preferable for assessing the future of an industry that is headed in many different directions at the same time. Predicting is appropriate for projecting the future of stable systems, while forecasting is the tool of choice for chaotic systems. Is health care today stable, or chaotic? You can skip the rest of this chapter if you think it is stable.

An everyday weather forecast nicely illustrates the fundamental concept of forecasting.[1] Meteorologists study how weather variables have interacted in the past, make adjustments for new factors, and then assign a probability to each possible outcome. (Consensus techniques and mathematical modeling are often used to incorporate new factors, such as global warming, into the calculation of a forecast's probabilities.) Hence, a 70 percent chance of rain implicitly means a 30 percent chance of all other weather possibilities. The forecast is right on target if seven-tenths of the forecast area gets rain and the other three-tenths does not.

Diversity is the Future

The paradoxical coexistence of two or more outcomes at the same time in the same system shows why forecasting is essential to our analysis of U.S. health care. In effect, *this book forecasts that 70 percent of providers will experience the end of real revenue growth by 2010.* The other 30 percent will experience something else. Their real revenues will continue to rise, thanks to circumstances like the good fortune to be in an exceptional market area or to have a source of income that is insulated from the changes in health care reimbursement (e.g., a trust fund, ownership of an oil well, royalties from a blockbuster drug, etc.). If the prediction were made that providers would see the end of revenue growth in 2010, at

---

1. Although the principal author (Bauer) is writing from his perspective of 35 years as a medical economist and health futurist, he was originally trained in meteorology and worked as a weatherman in Colorado in the 1960s. His next book will be an in-depth introduction to forecasting and other tools for being a health futurist.

least three in ten would question this prediction. And they would be correct to do so because it does not apply to them.

The difference between a forecast-based approach to the future, rich with perils and possibilities, and the standard practice of making predictions that put all providers in the same boat must be reiterated. The history of past predictions clearly supports a decision to forecast a range of simultaneous futures. Prospective payment, managed care, health maintenance organizations, the Clinton health plan, and tort reform are among the many trends that were widely predicted to define the health care system of the future. A few of these predictions affected some providers; others fizzled completely. Some played out in certain geographic markets and not at all in others.

Hospitals and medical groups will head in different directions because different forces are at play in different markets (geographic markets and product markets, in the relevant language of economic theory). Predictions that effectively dictate the same future for all providers inappropriately focus leaders on heading in one inescapable direction when they should be identifying and evaluating all possible directions. A forecast is much better for guiding an organization's approach to its future because it identifies choices to be made and actions that can be taken to influence the probabilities of desirable and undesirable possibilities.

The "Real" Meaning of This Forecast

Economists make an important distinction between nominal values and real values. Nominal values are measured in current dollars at a point in time; they are not adjusted for changes in the purchasing power of the money over time. Real values are adjusted for increases in the level of prices for goods and services bought with the money. For example, if a provider realizes a 5 percent growth in nominal revenue, the real value is 0 percent if the increase in costs of staying in business is also 5 percent. *Ceteris paribus* (all other things being equal), income is not *really* growing unless the increase in its nominal value is greater than the relevant rate of inflation. Likewise, net revenue stays the same when operating costs rise at the same rate as income in current dollars. Real revenue growth requires that nominal revenue rise more than nominal costs of doing business.

This book's forecast—70 percent of all providers will soon have no possibility of real revenue growth—means that increases in operating costs will be equal to or greater than revenue growth for the vast majority of health systems and medical groups. Simply put, their real revenue has peaked. Providers will have no ability to pass along increased operating costs to payers and patients. Trustees and chief executives of these organizations should be disturbed by this forecast and its implications. It means that the traditional methods for staying in business, raising prices and making better reimbursement arrangements with buyers, are finished.

Getting ahead by "business as usual" is impossible under such circumstances, and the chances of falling into a financial hole are increased. Economic theory offers two possible paths for decision makers to pursue. Either: 1) find ways to increase real revenues, which is not a viable plan for reasons presented in the rest of this chapter; or 2) find ways to be more efficient and effective so that existing resources can be reallocated to staying in business, which is the focus of the rest of this book. The majority of providers must quickly compensate for the end of increases in real revenue by harnessing waste and reallocating the savings to more productive use.

One final qualification about forecasts must be made. Even experienced forecasters accept the possibility that the future might hold a total surprise—an outcome that cannot be foreseen because it has never happened before. This "wild card" is sometimes called the GOK possibility, for "God only knows." For example, global warming is causing meteorologists to expand the GOK probability. The development of genetic and molecular medicine augurs similar possibilities for unknowable futures in health care. The "take-home" point: be prepared for some surprises. With this caveat, the following section discusses discernable trends that suggest most providers will soon find that their real revenues have peaked, even though demand has not.

The Precarious Economy

Providers, as a group, have grown accustomed to getting an ever-increasing share of the gross domestic product (GDP). American enterprise kept creating new wealth throughout the second half of the 20th century, and the health sector kept claiming just a little bit more of it every year. However, this era of good fortune is likely to end. Real economic growth is less certain than it has been at any time since the 1960s, and health care has lost much of the prestige and power that allowed it to grow at the expense of other sectors. Health care leaders are guilty of hubris if they believe that their share of the GDP pie will grow to 20 percent. (A more realistic assessment of economic forces suggests that providers should be pleased to keep the health sector's current share, around 17 percent. The current prospects for getting more are slim.)

A big part of the problem is the economy itself. As Alan Greenspan said in his final days as revered Chairman of the Federal Reserve System, nobody really knows how the economy works any more. It is full of surprises, which means that once-reliable principles for guiding the economy are suddenly producing unexpected and inexplicable results. For example, when this section was written during the last week of July, 2007, the stock market moved in one day from an all-time high to its worst loss in seven years—the same day that the government announced a five-fold increase in economic growth over the previous quarter. Stocks fell in value for companies that had announced good earnings, while share prices rose for a few big companies that had lost billions, but less than expected. Things were not making sense.

The financial news was filled with stories about investors "spooked" by the credit crisis and serious problems at some of the nation's leading hedge funds. CEOs of two Fortune 500 companies had just been given stiff prison sentences for their roles in bilking investors and deceiving auditors. High oil prices, a depressed housing sector, rising unemployment, global warming, and unfunded pension liabilities totaling hundreds of billions of dollars were also getting a lot of press. The mortgage industry was in shambles due to the cumulative effects of sub-prime lending, and the dollar had fallen to an all-time low against most major currencies. Interest rates started to rise much faster than usual, creating serious problems for health care organizations that had been making record investments in new campuses and new technologies because the costs of capital had been low for several years.

Some analysts might argue that this depiction sensationalizes the potential impact of these problems, but no one could argue that these circumstances are normal or predictable features of the economy that has been good to health care for several decades. As further evidence of disturbing changes in the way the economy works, predictions about the economy were hard to find during 2007.

Extrapolations from historical data were missing the mark. Analysts have even begun to think like forecasters, talking about the probabilities of the economy improving, stabilizing, or getting worse. The clear consensus was a rising likelihood that things were getting worse. More than one commentator was suggesting the light at the end of the tunnel just might be an oncoming train.

Under the circumstances, providers should not assume real revenues will rise in the future as they have in the past. Learning to get by with existing resources seems like the prudent plan. Becoming efficient and effective must become the new "business as usual." The risks of acting as if nothing has changed are enormous, especially for providers that borrow money in anticipation of rising real revenue.

Growing Competition for GDP

Health care's long-standing success at getting a bigger piece of the pie would be threatened for another reason, even if real GDP were to continue growing. In the past, nobody questioned the importance of paying for health care. The sector's position in the economy was sacrosanct. Of course, purchasers and policy makers have complained about the costs of health care, but spending on medical services almost always prevailed when union contracts had to be negotiated or government budgets had to be passed. The big cuts were made elsewhere because nothing was more important than health care—even though it was expensive. Now, health care has some detractors. People who defend the interests of other sectors are willing to fight health care in a zero-sum game.

Education is probably the most formidable competitor for available funds. Many thought leaders, notably Thomas Friedman in *The World is Flat*, make a strong case that inadequate investment in education is at or near the top of the list of reasons why the United States is declining. Elected officials at the state and local levels are beginning to put a much higher priority on education, at the expense of health care, in a growing number of jurisdictions. The need for massive investments in public infrastructure is also becoming obvious. Tragic dam breaks, bridge collapses, and failures of air traffic control are suddenly drawing attention to the woeful neglect in these critical areas. Last, and far from least, the looming costs of recovery from the wars in Iraq and Afghanistan are staggering.

Health care consequently has some formidable competition for a piece of the GDP, whether the pie grows or not. Providers can no longer assume that health care will be cut last or least when business and government allocate scarce resources. In addition, lobbyists for other interest groups may even speak ill of health care in battles for limited budgets. Becoming efficient and effective would be a splendid defense against intensifying claims that health care's prices are too high and its quality unacceptable.

International Challenges

Health industry analysts have always assumed that our medical economy was unaffected by international events. This assumption is not true today. The future of U.S. providers is definitely impacted by foreign factors beyond our control. For the first time, hospitals and medical groups need to take international considerations into account.

Economic globalization is arguably the international force with the most impact on health care. Offshore outsourcing has led to employment reductions in some major industries that traditionally provided health insurance to their workers. Immigration has a counterbalancing impact as foreign workers come to the United States and use health services here, but the net economic effect of outsourcing and immigration probably reduces the medical share of GDP. Rising foreign ownership of U.S. securities, particularly treasury certificates, increases both interest rates and market volatility. Neither outcome is beneficial to health care providers.

Of course, no one in the 20th century imagined that U.S. patients and their health care dollars would leave the country for hospital services, but "medical tourism" must now be taken seriously. Providers in foreign countries, aided by travel agencies and even some health insurers, are aggressively creating competitive opportunities for U.S. patients to go abroad. America's decline in medical research is also a factor that will cause health care to lose income. U.S. government policies toward stem-cell research, genetic therapies, and visas for foreign scientists have allowed other countries to become the world leaders in important domains of 21st century medicine. Many U.S. patients will travel abroad for health care, not to save money, but to get treatments that are unavailable here (with a resulting loss of revenue for domestic providers). Finally, charitable foundations in the United States are starting to spend tens of billions of dollars on health care projects in other countries. Health dollars that would have stayed here in the past are leaving the country.

New Competition for Traditional Business

New competitors will also reduce traditional providers' opportunities to increase their revenues. Even if year-to-year growth in real health spending were to continue, the incremental income would not necessarily go to hospitals and medical groups. National pharmacy chains and major retailers are entering the health care marketplace and competing for the same old dollars (i.e., not new dollars). They are aggressively building business in primary care, home health, specialty pharmacy, infusion therapy, and other medical services that do not need to be provided in a hospital or multiservice medical office building. For example, Wal-Mart and Walgreen's are opening nurse practitioner-staffed "convenience clinics" in their retail stores throughout the country. Their gain is almost certainly traditional providers' loss.

Consumerism, of course, is another major dimension of increasing competition for limited health care dollars. The topic has been treated extensively in recent years and requires no elaboration. Providers know they need to make changes as consumers become actively involved in deciding how their health care dollars will be spent. The important point is to take consumerism seriously. Private and public purchasers, health plans, consumer groups, and the media are all working to make consumers more cost conscious. The obvious intent of consumerism is to reduce spending on health care, creating one more way that providers' revenues could be capped.

Consumerism also illustrates the earlier point about complexity. Not all consumers will be informed and involved. Recent studies suggest that considerably fewer than half of all patients can reasonably be expected to use price and quality information to shop for health care anytime soon. However, even a relatively small contingent of savvy customers could be enough to divert revenue from traditional providers to the extent the consumers delay care due to "watchful waiting" or take their business to new retail clinics or to New Delhi.

Government Spending

Federal, state, and local governments currently pay half the money spent on health care in the United States. The future of providers' revenues correspondingly depends on the condition of the public purse. The prospects for additional spending are bleak at all three levels of government, beginning in Washington, D.C. Most of the 2008 presidential candidates promise a push toward universal access if elected, but child health insurance is the only program for which more money is possible. The chances for any other federal increases are extremely low, given economic instability and rising interest rates (i.e., the rising costs of financing federal debt to increase spending on health care).

Even if universal access were to be implemented within the next few years, most of the newly insured—people who don't have health insurance now because they don't have any extra money to spend—would have high deductible and/or minimum-coverage health plans. Hospitals and physicians would be trading a headache for an upset stomach. Medicare's looming expenditures for baby boomers are also a brake on new spending, at the same time other public needs (e.g., education, defense, infrastructure) are rising in priority. Finally, the IRS is pushing nonprofit hospitals to give away more care to justify their tax exemptions. The health care industry will be lucky if the federal government maintains current levels of health spending. Real increases are almost unimaginable.

The prospects for more government spending on health care are at least as grim at the state and local levels. The unfunded pension liabilities for relatively old public workforces are staggering. For example, New Jersey has a $58 billion exposure for health care alone, and 40 percent of all state employees are eligible to retire within next 10 years. New York and California have nearly equal unfunded liabilities. Consequently, analysts foresee some economic disasters on the horizon as local governments fail to meet their pension obligations. Speaking of disasters, local governments are paying the price of recovering from hurricanes, fires, floods, and droughts because the federal government has not made extra funds available as promised. States also face the financial burdens of renewing National Guard units incapacitated by the wars in Iraq and Afghanistan. More state and local money for health care? "Fuhgeddaboudit," as they say in New Jersey.

Supply and Demand

A brief review of supply and demand provides a fitting bridge between this chapter's review of economic problems and the remaining chapters' focus on solutions. As everyone learned in basic economics classes, markets work well when supply and demand are in equilibrium. Unfortunately, just about all the evidence suggests the market is not balanced and even moving toward greater imbalance.

This chapter has focused on limits to payment for care. Unfortunately, limiting payment does not necessarily limit demand. All other things being equal, a serious economic problem occurs when buyers' demand rises and sellers' income does not. Several trends suggest a dramatic increase in unfunded or underfunded demands that will be placed on providers in the near future. The problems posed through demand by baby boomers are already well known, as are the potential costs of caring for retirees whose health benefits were terminated by their employers.

The less-publicized problems of a few other groups could be just as serious. For example, soldiers returning from

Iraq and Afghanistan will have almost unimaginable needs for a wide range of health services. Congress has not given the Veterans Health Administration enough money to meet this demand; therefore many soldiers will show up at civilian hospitals. Even more unpaid demand will be generated by the thousands of injured civilian contractors who are returning to the United States without any coverage to pay for their care. Finally, the number of insured patients with exclusions for pre-existing conditions will also grow as a result of mobility in the labor force.

The supply picture looks equally as negative. The number of physicians in many specialties, especially primary care, is inadequate to meet today's or tomorrow's needs. Nurses, pharmacists, therapists, and other allied health professionals are also in persistently and seriously short supply. The situation can only deteriorate over the next few years because academic health centers have not been able to expand their training programs. Finally, the physical plant of many provider facilities has reached its limits—not necessarily in size, but rather in capacity to house the technologies and teams of modern medicine.

Obviously, this review suggests that demand is likely to swamp supply. However, as already shown, the increase in demand is not likely to be accompanied by more real money. Providers will try to increase their supply of medical services because meeting demand is a proud pillar of professionalism in health care, but 70 percent will find the task impossible. With no more money to pay the costs of more demand, most providers will face two options: 1) bankruptcy, with liquidation every bit as possible as reorganization, or 2) find ways to provide more with less. The good news is that economic theory and real-world examples show that the second choice is possible. The remaining chapters explain how.

| TWO |

THE ECONOMIC IMPERATIVE: EFFICIENCY (COST)

Health care is not the first U.S. industry in which most producers have had to change their way of doing business in order to survive. Indeed, it may be among the last. Dramatic changes in the marketplace have forced almost every other sector of the economy to restructure over the past two decades. Today's leading airlines, banks, accounting firms, manufacturers, entertainment groups, insurers, retailers, and energy distributors bear little resemblance to the companies that dominated their respective industries in the 1980s and 1990s. Many businesses changed their names to reflect major reorganization and reorientation. Others kept their well-established corporate identities but shifted to very different business models and value propositions.

Basic principles of economics are behind the successful, *enduring* transformations in other industries. Some infamous enterprises like Enron and WorldCom used noneconomic methods to grow impressively for a while, but persistent investigative reporters and dedicated federal prosecutors ultimately ended the run of companies that resorted to fraud and greed. Gaming the system is a temporary solution at best and a crime at worst. Following good business practices is the reliable way to stay in business. This analysis assumes that successful health care providers will transform legally and ethically.

Ethical managers who successfully overcame the challenges of change in nonhealth industries consistently returned to fundamental principles they learned in Economics 101. They examined every aspect of producing and selling their product, constantly pursuing ways to do things differently because business as usual did not look promising. One universal ingredient in the "secret sauce" of their successful economic transformations is operational awareness of the time frames in which changes can be made.

Short-Run Versus Long-Run

Basic principles of economics are often forgotten, probably because they are poorly taught at the introductory level and never truly understood. Consequently, successful transformation of health care delivery organizations begins with a quick review of one of the most important foundations of economic analysis—the difference between short-run and long-run perspectives. Hospital executives and medical group leaders must incorporate this difference in their thinking as they respond to new threats in the medical marketplace.

As economists say, with their proclivity for understatement, the difference between the short-run and the long-run is not trivial. Successful executives understand the important difference between short-run and long-run perspectives. They see the need for short-run and long-run solutions to problems that are threatening the enterprise, and they manage them as distinctly different tasks. Conversely, inquests into business failures almost always find that managers focused on one perspective at the expense of the other.

Neither time frame is defined in economic analysis as a specific interval on a calendar. Measuring the short-run as one year and the long-run as three years is a common practice, but it misses the critical point of applied economic analysis.

- The **short-run** is the period when inputs cannot be changed. The manager's task is to find the best combination of existing inputs (e.g., employees on the payroll, supplies in the stockroom) to produce a desired good or service. The quantities of all resources are fixed in the short run. The only approach to improved performance is trying different combinations of the resources at hand.

- The **long-run** begins when all inputs can be changed. The manager's task in the long run is to evaluate alternative combinations of inputs and to make trade-offs that will produce better goods and services. All resources are variable in the long run, so old resources can be replaced with new ones in pursuit of a strong corporate future.

Leaders who have successfully transformed other industries all made the jump from short-run to long-run thinking. After fine-tuning the interaction of existing inputs to address immediate problems, they learned how to rethink products and production processes. They envisioned not only different ways to run the day-to-day businesses, but also the possibility of doing new things that had promising prospects for success once they had negotiated the necessary trade-offs—selling a unit, developing a new product, reengineering a process, retraining employees, outsourcing a business function, creating a partnership (sometimes with a competitor), and so forth.

Health care executives need to accomplish the same transition in shaping the future of their enterprises. Responding to the medical marketplace's new imperatives requires long-run thinking where everything can be changed. Tasks can be reassigned to new personnel. Procedures can be revised. Space can be remodeled to serve different purposes. Hospitals and physicians can work for the same economic enterprise. In operational terms, the ability to identify feasible alternatives and to make responsive changes is a critical success factor for the future.

Tactics Versus Strategy

Academic observers have often said that economists and business school professors teach similar concepts but present them in different terms. Back in their student days, aspiring health care executives had to decide whether or not this difference was important when they made the educational choice between a master's degree in health administration (MHA) and a master's degree in business administration (MBA), often with a health care emphasis.

Readers with MHA degrees should be familiar with the difference between the short-run and long-run because they took courses taught by economists with PhDs. This economic terminology may be unfamiliar to those who studied health care management at a business school, where professors with DBAs talked in terms of tactics and strategy when addressing managerial flexibility over time.

- **Tactics** is the realm of management skills necessary for dealing with the short-run. In effect, department heads need to be tacticians. They work with limited budgets (i.e., fixed resources) that define the personnel and materials available for doing a specific job in a fixed period of time. In fact, efforts to change inputs and processes at the department level in a fiscal year are generally counterproductive for the enterprise because departments are highly interdependent. Unbudgeted change that solves problems in one department almost always causes problems in another.

- **Strategy** is the realm of management skills needed for structuring proactive, enterprise-wide responses to anticipated changes in the marketplace. C-suite executives should predominantly be strategists, with the ability to delegate tactics to trusted and talented subordinates. Chief executives need to be long-run thinkers who explore alternatives within and across departments. They need to have the skills *and courage* to reallocate internal resources to achieve better outcomes in response to meaningful trends in the marketplace.

Business school professors use a variety of examples to illustrate the operationally meaningful difference between tactics and strategy. In sports, coaches are the tacticians because they must try to win with the players who suited up for each game. Team owners are the strategists who decide whether to trade players or get a new coach so that future games will be played differently. In the military, lieutenants are the tacticians responsible for fighting with the troops and armaments that are on the field for a given battle. Generals make strategic decisions, such as shifting resources between naval, air, and ground troops. Their reallocations will change the way future battles are fought.

This book is written principally for health care's counterparts of team owners (trustees) and generals (senior executives, both managerial and clinical). Of course, these leaders must have the courage and the skills to rally the troops once the strategic decisions have been made—as abundantly illustrated in the following pages with practical examples from health care delivery organizations that have strengthened their organizations by setting new directions and motivating stakeholders to move cooperatively toward these destinations.

Challenge for Success: Long-Run Strategy

Given the marketplace's new imperatives, leaders of successful hospitals and medical groups will need to be long-run strategists. They will integrate the professional economist's constant evaluation of variability in all resources with the business professor's persistent responsiveness to anticipated changes in the marketplace. Their decisions and actions will reflect an often-quoted but seldom honored maxim: if you don't like what you've always gotten, quit doing what you've always done. Doing things differently will be a key to success for most trustees and executives.

Although this book presents many successful examples of future-focused change, it assumes that long-run strategists are uncommon in hospitals and medical groups. The norm in health care is leadership that intentionally chooses to conduct business as usual. Many trustees, senior executives, and clinical leaders do not want to assume the responsibilities and risks of being a long-run strategist. For a variety of reasons, intentional and unintentional, they choose not to rock the boat. They are dedicated and honorable people, but they are not interested in "breaking eggs to make an omelet.[1]"

Why protect the *status quo*? Most health care leaders do not want to experience the predictably unpleasant consequences of terminating a marginal service line, assigning employees to unfamiliar tasks, confronting a "my way or the highway" member of the medical staff, collaborating with the hospital down the street, or standing up to a powerful third party that has an unfair advantage in the marketplace. Managing by conflict avoidance was generally not fatal to the enterprise when purchasers and payers could ultimately be counted on to pay the high costs of the resulting inefficiencies.

However, as discussed in the previous chapter, third parties are no longer able and/or willing to subsidize waste in health care. And consumers definitely do not have the inclination—even if they have the money—to pay their rising share of the bill for services priced above perceived value. Unless providers have a generous and forgiving benefactor, a large and

---

1. We received strong statements about this point when we asked health care executives to comment on our book proposal. Many respondents suggested that our analysis and recommendations would be poorly received by the large number of CEOs who are within a few years of retirement. Most of these "fifty-something" executives would understand the need for dramatic change in their organizations, but they would not willingly rise to the strategic challenges of managing change so late in their careers. Our informal poll did not have the methodological power to prove the point, but the consistency of responses from independent commentators suggests a problem worthy of further consideration. Under such circumstances, trustees will face an unpleasant choice between the organization's need to change sooner rather than later and a valued chief executive's desire to maintain stability for a few more years. Creative solutions must be crafted on a case-by-case basis because trustees are ultimately expected to act in the best interests of the organization, not the CEO. Ironically, a CEO who does not want to shake things up in the final years of a career may actually be the best person to do it because he or she has nothing to lose (e.g., no need for a good reference for the next move up the ladder).

unrestricted endowment, or exceptional market power, they must implement strategies for long-run change in the way they produce medical services. They must control operating costs because they cannot make real (i.e., inflation-adjusted) revenue rise. In a word, providers must become efficient.

E-Imperative #1: Efficiency

Imagine a pop quiz where health care leaders, politicians, and policy analysts are asked to define *efficiency* in economic terms and to describe a process for improving the efficiency of a medical service. As a rule, answers would be highly variable. This inconsistency points to a serious problem: the health industry is not efficient because its leaders do not have a common understanding of efficiency and efficient production processes.

The problem has become so pervasive and its consequences so expensive that correcting it is an essential precondition for meaningful improvements in the U.S. health care delivery system. The current debate over health reform is focused almost exclusively on the uninsured, but inefficiency in provider organizations is the elephant in the living room that everyone ignores. Even if all Americans acquired health insurance, the United States would still have an unaffordable health care system, as long as providers lack the knowledge, authority, responsibility, and/or incentives to become efficient.

Consequently, *a common operational understanding of efficiency and its processes must be created across the industry as a precondition for providing affordable health care of acceptable quality.* Real progress toward these fundamental goals of health reform cannot occur until "everyone is singing off the same page." The good news is that economists (and management engineers, who apply the same principles) have a standardized definition of efficiency and a common set of quantitative tools for determining the most efficient combination of resources needed to produce a specific good or service. Their concept of efficiency is, metaphorically speaking, an excellent page from which all should be singing.

The next section tells health care leaders what they need to know in order to articulate strategies for becoming efficient. The nitty-gritty tasks of implementing strategies should be delegated to managers and consultants who have spent years learning and using the tools of the efficiency trade. Leaders responsible for their organization's future only need to understand the fundamental concepts and why efficiency is quickly becoming essential to the success of their organizations. They do not need to know how to do it.

Executive-Level Briefing on Efficiency

In the theory of economics and the models of management engineering, *efficiency* is defined in two different, but equivalent, ways:

- **Maximum output for a fixed budget**—An outcome where managers have determined the combination of inputs that produces the greatest quantity of a good or service for a given amount of money (for example, finding the combination of nurses, physicians, treatment spaces, and technologies that yields the maximum number of annual visits to an emergency department for an annual operating budget of 5 million dollars). From this perspective, efficiency is the highest output you can produce for a specific number of dollars.

or

- **Minimum cost for a fixed output**—An outcome where managers have determined the combination of inputs that produces a fixed quantity of a good or service at the least-expensive cost (for example, finding the lowest annual budget that is needed to buy the resources necessary to produce 50,000 annual visits to an emergency department). From this perspective, efficiency is the minimum number of dollars needed to meet a predetermined production goal.

Most people are surprised that one question can require two answers to be correct. (This uncommon duality would partly explain the wide variation in answers to the hypothetical pop-quiz question. Nearly everyone would provide only one answer, which means that nearly everyone would be half-right at best.) Even more surprising, the two answers seem to be very different, but in reality, they are only different ways to describe the same point—the bottoms of various configurations of the U-shaped cost curves that college students learned about in Economics 101.

In order to tell leaders only what they need to know, the authors have intentionally (even mercifully?) decided not to clutter this book with several pages of U-shaped cost curves and explanations of production functions. Anyone who really wants a refresher can get it from a basic economics textbook, but a health care executive cannot move his or her organization forward by using U-shaped cost curves in presentations to stakeholders or discussions with managers. Besides, the experts who are actually going to do the work will already know the underlying concepts and related mathematics. Executives need to know that efficiency can be achieved by following one of two different paths—minimizing costs for a predetermined output or maximizing output for a predetermined budget.

Problems to Avoid

Three serious mistakes are commonly made in pursuit of efficiency. To avoid one or more of these traps, leaders of health care delivery organizations must understand the potential pitfalls of efficiency projects and communicate them to line managers who are responsible for translating long-run strategy into practice. If there were going to be a pop quiz at the end of this chapter, the exam would definitely include questions on all three points.

First, efficiency in any production unit (e.g., a medical group department or a hospital service line) can be pursued one way *or* the other, but not both ways at once. A common mistake is to define efficiency as the greatest output for the least cost. The coexistence of a maximum (greatest output) and a minimum (least cost) in a closed system is mathematically impossible. As MHA and MBA students should have learned in their quantitative methods courses, only one variable can be maximized or minimized in a system with limited resources—the market situation that health care is now entering. Other factors can serve as constraints (i.e., the fixed limits on the values of key parameters), which is why efficiency is defined either as cost minimization for a fixed output or output maximization for a fixed cost.

Second, managers must decide, or be told, which of these two paths to follow in pursuit of the efficient outcome for their departments or service lines. Production units are often told to produce more for less, a dictum that almost always promotes inefficiency because it does not force managers to focus on doing one thing as well as possible. Instead, they should start with an output objective, such as the number of services to be provided in a unit, or an annual budget. Department heads, with support of efficiency experts, as needed, should then evaluate different input combinations that would minimize cost to meet the fixed output goal or maximize output to stay within the fixed budget. Output maximization is not inherently better than cost minimization. The enterprise's financial status will usually suggest which approach to take, with the possibility of case-by-case differences. The senior executive's task is to make sure that line managers focus on one approach or the other, not both, when they adopt efficiency as a core organizational value.

Third, efficiency is a moving target in health care. Holding steadfastly to an efficient outcome can prove counterproductive. Scientific advances force new clinical demands on providers, faster than ever before, and new technologies constantly expand the realm of possibilities for maximizing outputs or minimizing costs. A combination of health professionals, equipment, and space that is efficient today could quickly become inefficient upon the publication of new clinical evidence, introduction of better technology, or a change in the payment for care. Rapidity of change reinforces the compelling need for executives to take a long-run strategic view of their enterprises. They must propagate the view that all resources are variable and ensure that appropriate trade-offs are constantly made within their enterprises. Measurable movement in the direction of efficiency is generally the best that can be expected under the circumstances. Consequently, processes for becoming efficient receive major attention throughout the rest of this book.

The Bottom Line: Waste

One single word translates the theoretical concept of efficiency into the operational reality of provider organizations: *waste*. Inefficiency, the "other side of the (efficiency) coin," is waste. Consequently, efficiency and waste are inversely related. Efficiency decreases as waste increases, and vice versa. Another important dimension of waste is opportunity costs—the other things that could be produced with the same resources.

Efficiency experts define waste as resources consumed in excess of those needed to minimize costs of a specified output or to maximize output for a specified budget. To extend an earlier example, assume a management engineering study determines that a maximum of 50,000 visits of acceptable quality could be provided in a particular hospital's emergency department (ED) for an annual budget of $4,000,000. One million dollars is being wasted if the hospital is actually spending $5,000,000 to deliver 50,000 ED visits.

The wasted $1,000,000 could include money spent on overstaffing that causes nurses to get in each other's way when the ED is busy (diminishing returns, in economic terms). It could be the cumulative costs of $100-an-hour physicians waiting a few minutes here and a few minutes there for $15-an-hour technicians to assist with procedures, or the salaries of several clerks who are needed to write information on paper forms and keyboard the same information into electronic databases.

Drug administration errors would likely account for part of the wasted million, as would the cost of redundant diagnostic tests to get information that was already in a patient's medical record—inaccessibly located elsewhere in the hospital. Waste would include money spent on duplicative diagnostics, where a radiologist or a pathologist repeats a review of test results interpreted hours earlier by the ED physician. From the perspective of an efficiency expert, it could also be the cost of supplies discarded because they were stored beyond the expiration date or opened but not used. Waste can even be money spent to build more ED treatment areas because housekeepers are not always available to clean bays as soon as patients are transferred elsewhere.

Comparable examples of inefficiency exist across the board in almost all provider organizations. To keep our analysis simple and focused, this chapter is not padded with lots of specific examples. Readers understand the general point: hospitals, medical groups, and other provider organizations are inefficient. Capturing wasted resources and reallocating them to more important use is imperative because purchasers are not going to keep paying more for medical care.

How Much Waste in Health Care?

Is there enough waste in provider organizations to justify formal programs for capturing and reallocating it? If wasted resources were harnessed, would the recovered money offset the incremental revenue that will *not* be coming from purchasers, payers, and patients? Obviously, long-run strategies to become efficient will themselves be wasteful if they cost more than they yield. Becoming efficient must improve "cash flow." It will not be worth the time and effort if the sums to be reallocated are small.

Almost everyone who has worked in a hospital or medical group will agree that providers are extremely inefficient (i.e., wasteful). Several widely published studies, well known to anyone who attends national meetings or reads trade journals, have produced sobering numbers. Estimates of waste range between one-fifth (20 percent) and one-third (33 percent) of national health care expenditures. These studies have not focused on inefficiency by type of provider, but approximately 60 percent of our health care dollars goes to hospitals and physicians. Adjusting the estimates of system-wide waste by this factor, inferred waste in hospitals and medical groups collectively ranges between 12 percent and 18 percent of dollars spent on health care.

Because a substantial portion of total waste occurs outside hospitals and medical groups, specifically in the reimbursement system (a problem addressed at the end of the book), providers should not extrapolate numbers from the health system as a whole to their organizations. Once again, leaders are urged to avoid general statements in health care and to assess the prospects for efficiency from the specific perspective of their own organizations. A few health systems probably do waste as much as one-third of their resources. At the other extreme, a few exemplary organizations have already eliminated the waste in operations. The vast majority lies somewhere in between, arguably capable of making long-run strategic changes that could liberate between 12 percent and 18 percent of the annual spending on hospital and physician services for more productive use. Reallocating this much money to productive uses is worth the time and effort.

International comparisons provide further evidence of significant waste in U.S. health care. Among the world's industrialized countries, the United States is effectively at the top of the list in spending on medical services and at the bottom of the list in producing health for its population. These comparative data do not prove that any given provider organization is wasteful. However, they strongly suggest waste in the system as a whole because other countries get proportionally much more health from the money they spend on health care.

From the perspective of efficiency, health policy analysts should estimate how much more health could be produced for 17 percent of the gross domestic product (through reallocation of wasted resources within health care) *or* how much less GDP could be spent to produce current levels of health (with wasted resources removed from health care). This approach would be more productive than the current focus on reforming health care through universal access. Five percent of GDP would be a defensible "ballpark" estimate of the difference between health expenditures in the United States and comparable countries—and a reasonable estimate of waste that could be reallocated or eliminated from this perspective. Reallocation within health care is strongly defended in the policy recommendations at the end of this book.

Finally, the process of conducting the research for this book produced compelling supportive evidence from delivery organizations that have gone from multimillion dollar losses to strong operating margins within a year or two of focusing on efficiency and effectiveness (see Chapter 3). Stories of these successes are the case studies in the following chapters. Economic theory is often criticized for being unrelated to economic practice, but some remarkable turnarounds show that efficiency is a critical success factor in the real world of health care in the early 21st century. Capturing, retaining, and reallocating waste will be the key to survival and growth for nearly all providers.

| THREE |

THE CLINICAL IMPERATIVE: EFFECTIVENESS (QUALITY)

Efficiency is not the only performance measure on which health care lags behind almost all other U.S. industries. Providers of medical services also have a general reputation of being ineffective. To survive in highly competitive markets where the overall quality of products has become as important as the costs of producing them, leading companies in nonhealth sectors of the economy have been forced to become effective—to tell customers what to expect and to deliver as promised.

Effectiveness is not the same thing as efficiency. The common practice of using *efficiency* and *effectiveness* as synonyms is wrong and misleading. Businesses in a particular industry can be efficient and ineffective or inefficient and effective. For example, Japanese cars were sold at remarkably low prices when introduced to the U.S. market in the 1960s because they were produced efficiently (i.e., cheaply). These imports quickly developed a reputation for poor performance and low quality. They were ineffective products. Japanese automakers did not originally give U.S. consumers what was expected in an automobile. Cars from Japan sold poorly and became the metaphor for shoddy goods, even though they were relatively inexpensive.

Clearly, the current situation is quite different. Japanese companies ultimately focused intense efforts on producing a car that would appeal to the U.S. motorist. In less than two decades, they set and met standards that established their "foreign" cars as best buys in the U.S. automobile market. ("Foreign" is in quotes because Japanese auto makers also became efficient by assembling many of their cars in the United States, thus avoiding high costs for transporting finished automobiles across the Pacific Ocean. Ironically, the consultants who taught them how to master efficiency and effectiveness were Americans...but that's another story.)

Effectiveness: Compliance with Specifications of Performance

The basic concept is simple. Effectiveness is a measure of the relative compliance with objective specifications of expected performance. If a good or service does everything that it was designed to do, it is 100 percent effective (regardless of its cost of production or price). If it performs below specified expectations, it is correspondingly less effective. Take, for example, a robotic drug dispensing system that is designed to fill 1,000 prescriptions every hour. If it only fills 900 prescriptions per hour once installed in your organization, the device is 90 percent effective because it is achieving only 90 percent of its promised performance.

Leaders who do not remember studying effectiveness in Economics 101 will probably remember studying the concept in an introductory statistics course. Most statistics textbooks have a problem set where a random sample of a product (e.g., a light bulb) is selected off the assembly line, the items in the sample are tested, and the number of defective products in the sample is compared statistically with the number of defects allowed by the production specifications. An equation extrapolates the sample test results to the entire production run, incorporating the desired level of confidence in the results. The batch is accepted if the rate of defects is below a predetermined threshold defined as effectiveness in production. If the number of defects exceeds the threshold of statistical significance, the production process is reengineered.

The basic statistical methods for judging actual performance against specified performance are generally categorized under the heading of process improvement techniques. Management by objectives, Six Sigma, total quality management (TQM), and lean manufacturing are familiar examples of techniques used to improve production processes. The tools of process improvement are usually designed to cut waste and to produce better products. They nicely encompass both efficiency and effectiveness. (See Chapter 6 for an executive-level exploration of these techniques and their applications in health care delivery organizations.)

Neither Cost Nor Value

In models of consumer economics and production engineering, effectiveness is a particularly important consideration at the interface between customers' expectations and producers' promises. Consumers and producers both want effective products. For example, if an automobile conforms with the manufacturer's specifications—it really gets 32 miles per gallon and goes 100,000 miles without any major repairs, as advertised—the car is an effective product to the company that made it and to the customer who bought it. Neither the buyer nor the seller incurs any unexpected expenses or unpleasant surprises. Effective products clearly help create consumer satisfaction and product loyalty—valuable "blue sky" assets for any seller.

The automaker's cost of producing the car is not included in the measurement of effectiveness. A car that meets all expectations could be produced efficiently or inefficiently. Effectiveness is not determined by the purchase price, either. A dealer's markup (cleverly disguised as a discount off the Manufacturer Suggested Retail Price, or MSRP) doesn't impact the car's mileage, service record, comfort, safety, or other performance measures. To prove the point, someone can buy both a lemon from a high-priced auto dealer with a gleaming showroom near an upscale mall or a completely satisfactory car from a guy in a plaid suit at a lot on the rundown side of town. Experience shows that an expensive product does not necessarily meet expectations, and an inexpensive product can exceed them.

The subjective relationship between price and consumer satisfaction is value. It has nothing to do with effectiveness (or efficiency, for that matter). Value will be extremely important to the success of hospitals and medical groups in the new marketplace. However, *health care delivery organizations must master efficiency and effectiveness before they can produce true value.* Real value cannot exist if products are overpriced or underperforming. Value-based purchasers in competitive markets want to know what they can reasonably expect for their money. Some health care providers get it backwards, trying to sell value without first doing the hard work of defining effective services and producing them efficiently. This approach will be increasingly unproductive as the medical marketplace becomes more competitive.

Why Effectiveness Is an Imperative

The effectiveness imperative for executives and trustees ensures that their health care delivery organizations do the right things in the right order. *To be effective, providers must begin by defining precise specifications of the good or service they are going to produce.* In other words, the first step for any provider organization that aspires to be demonstrably effective—a critical success factor in competitive, accountable, and resource-limited industries—is to state objective criteria against which performance will be measured before production begins. Only then can resources be allocated and managed to meet the performance objectives. Effectiveness defined after production is completed is meaningless.

Getting graded in college is a useful analogy because hospitals and medical groups are starting to receive a lot of grades. A grade should objectively measure a student's effectiveness in meeting a course's objectives. Students rightly resent professors who do not announce the criteria for grading before (and often after) a test is taken—especially when they put a lot of work into answers that seemed important to them but apparently did not impress the professor. On the other hand, teachers with clear grading policies are respected, because students can do their work with advance knowledge of how it will be judged. Hospitals and medical groups can reap comparable benefits by announcing objective criteria for grading before their work is put to the test.

Beyond serving as a foundation for assessment of current performance, measures of effectiveness also define the long-run destination for a clinical enterprise. They establish the level of performance that will be used to grade the organization's output of goods and services in the future. Therefore, directors and senior executives have a strategic responsibility to commit their organization to measurable effectiveness. They can initiate reallocation of resources as needed to hold the enterprise accountable to specified levels of performance. Conversely, if leaders with strategic responsibility do not issue a system-wide mandate for effectiveness, the action surely will not be taken by anyone else.

Once top leadership has adopted effectiveness as a strategic imperative for the entire enterprise, managers must have the tactical responsibility and authority to meet the measurable objectives of performance. Again, an analogy helps to illustrate the point. A strategic leader in a health care delivery organization is like a visionary architect who creates the concept drawings that are entered in a competition for a building project. The provider's department managers are like the engineers and designers who prepare the blueprints and the workers who do the construction for the architect whose concept is selected. The final result is best when the strategists are responsible for defining and enforcing vision and the tacticians for organizing and executing performance. In other words, top-level leaders must clearly communicate an orientation to effectiveness in the organizational vision that line managers are responsible for actualizing.

Effectiveness and Quality in Health Care

Effectiveness in health care delivery can be assessed by several nonmonetary measures. (By definition, money is not a valid measure of effectiveness. Cost in dollars is a defining measure of efficiency, not effectiveness.) Consumers might judge the effectiveness of providers on the basis of waiting time, personalization of service, or convenience of location. Providers might use accreditation, public designations (e.g.,

"100 top" status), or market share to judge their own effectiveness. Buyers and sellers do not necessarily use the same criteria to measure effectiveness, a point commonly made by automobile industry analysts.

Fortunately, quality of care is rapidly emerging as a common standard for measuring effectiveness in the medical marketplace. Quality is not the only criterion that consumers and providers might agree to use to measure effectiveness, but it is probably the one that has the most appeal to all concerned—especially in a business that makes the difference between life and death and consumes one-sixth of our gross domestic product. Quality stands as the fundamental criterion that should be used to measure effectiveness in the U.S. health care delivery system. (In the same impish spirit that national public radio's Michael Feldman tells *Whad'Ya Know?* listeners to get their own radio show if they do not like the answers to his quiz questions, readers can write their own book if they think something else is more important than quality in responding to the effectiveness imperative.)

Quality is, therefore, the centerpiece of this book's prescriptions for providers' responses to the effectiveness imperative. Concepts like value and consumer satisfaction play important supporting roles, but quality must trump all other considerations when strategic choices need to be made in health care delivery organizations. Quality should not be compromised for potential gains in other dimensions of effectiveness. Effectiveness-cum-quality is what consumers are coming to expect most from providers. Last, and definitely not least, professionalism compels providers to defend quality as the #1 criterion for gauging their work. Quality is the 21st century embodiment of Hippocrates' enduring challenge to health professionals, "First, do no harm."

Clarifying the Meaning of Quality

For quality to become the common and preferred measure of effectiveness in health care, it must have a consistent definition. The concept as currently applied is too nebulous to be operationally useful. The word, *quality*, undoubtedly appears in the mission statement of every hospital and medical group in the country. Yet, enormous regional and local variations abound in the processes and outcomes of care. The quality of medical care in the United States clearly runs the gamut from excellent to abysmal. (Indeed, some hospitals provide the best of care and the worst of care on any given day.) If all the providers in the country can lay claim to producing "quality" health care, then the word as currently used is meaningless. It cannot be a differentiator when it encompasses everything.

Fortunately, some progressive delivery systems and professional organizations from all around the country—many of them featured as case studies in this book—are beginning to create a consensus approach for defining quality in ways that would allow it to be a valid (i.e., meaningful) and reliable (i.e., accurate) measure of effectiveness. The common denominator of this progressive movement is consistent use of measurable, clinically proven standards for evaluating the continuum of processes involved in delivery of medical services.

Quality health care is becoming *quantified* health care. In response to the imperatives of the new medical marketplace, progressive providers are learning how to define quality numerically, not verbally. Ironically, in a semantic twist, quality as the measure of effectiveness in health care must be defined quantitatively—not qualitatively. The structure and process descriptions of traditional accreditation mechanisms (e.g., committees that meet weekly and review selected cases) are not adequate for the new task. Hospitals and medical groups must produce honest numbers to support pre-specified claims of providing quality care. Without supportive data, the typical mission statement's words about quality will be meaningless.

An organization's leaders must respond to the effectiveness imperative by adopting policies that impose quantitative approaches to measuring and managing quality at all stages of operations. The strategic plan must be updated to force the enterprise to shift the nature of its stated quality commitment from rhetorically subjective (e.g., "We work as a team to be as good as possible.") to accountably objective (e.g., "We meet specific, published performance standards in all that we do."). As more provider organizations make this necessary shift, the definition of quality will evolve from a philosophical concept to a data-driven process. Executive-level summaries of these processes are presented in Chapter 6.

Limitations of Historical Efforts

Quality has been a major concern since the 1960s when Professor Avedis Donabedian established structure, process, and outcomes as the standard measures for grading and comparing health care delivery systems. Safety was added to the list of qualitative criteria during the 1990s. The Joint Commission for Accreditation of Health Care Organizations (JCAHO), other industry accrediting groups, and government regulatory agencies continually refined their methods for evaluating providers on the basis of these four criteria. Compliance with standards and regulations was deemed to be an adequate proxy for the quality of a provider's health services.

However, several well-publicized studies by the Institute of Medicine (IOM) and other independent research organizations demonstrated that providers were not producing a consistently good product. Hundreds of thousands of avoidable deaths and injuries were directly attributed to flaws in the processes for producing health care. Decades of self-enforcement through accreditation have not ensured the production of truly effective health services. In response, groups of experts have promulgated several dozen quality indicators over the past decade and used them to link reimbursement with performance. Meeting the standards is rewarded with a small bonus, but not meeting them is not punished.

Although a laudable move in a desirable direction, pay for performance (P4P) is not without serious flaws. Many of the quality indicators have been criticized for insensitivity to clinically significant differences in patients who have the same general diagnosis. For example, 100 percent compliance with the standard for administering aspirin to all patients with myocardial infarction does not produce quality medical care for patients who should not receive aspirin. Some patients are harmed by compliance with the quality indicator, even though the provider's bottom line is helped via P4P.

Consequently, respected clinical journals have published many letters and editorials that identify serious problems created by the P4P solution. The conflicts will undoubtedly be resolved over time, but disease-specific quality indicators cannot be expected to produce needed improvements fast enough to help providers survive the impending limits in real revenue growth. Bonus payments for performance are "a drop in the bucket" compared to total resources that providers will need to stay in business. Also, the most likely result of pay for performance is nonpayment for nonperformance. Effectiveness is all the more imperative.

Effectiveness Comes from Within

Partisan gridlock and more pressing financial obligations will prevent governments from solving the problems. Likewise, the health care industry itself will not produce timely solutions due to its internal divisions, intense competition, and related issues of antitrust law. Providers waiting for someone else to give them a fair and fast financial fix only delude themselves because almost all consumers with financial resources can go elsewhere for their health care. Clearly, the limited success of collective efforts to improve quality over the past 40 years suggests that hospitals and medical groups will need to become effective on their own, one provider at a time.

Quality indicators can provide a desirable goal for a provider's production processes when appropriately adjusted to reflect clinically significant differences in patients with the same medical problem. However, quality indicators and production goals do not include useful information on how to reach them. Hospitals and medical groups need to have and follow operational procedures that produce the desired results. They need specific instructions on how to get where they need to go. The positive news is that health care providers can adopt production systems from other industries that have already overcome their own financial crises by becoming efficient and effective.

Therefore, health care's "take-home" lesson from other industries is that organizations must implement specific production processes in order to meet predetermined criteria of effectiveness and other performance indicators established by regulators or the marketplace. Objective, data-driven goals will not be met simply because they exist. Becoming effective requires more than finding new production processes that are appropriate to the task. It also requires making an enterprise-wide commitment to using the new processes all the time.

Understanding and applying this lesson is one of the most important contributions that a trustee or senior executive can make to a successful future for his or her organization. Setting and meeting objective measures of performance is the key to survival in the emerging medical marketplace where nobody is willing to pay more for what they get and everybody can go somewhere else for what they want. To paraphrase a statement often made about a treasured pastime, like fishing or golf, "Becoming an effective health care delivery organization is not a matter of life and death. It's more important than that."

Pursuing Efficiency and Effectiveness Together

Really astute readers have probably foreseen the possibility of an inconsistency in this analysis. This book makes compelling arguments for efficiency and effectiveness, which might give the impression that it will now claim that hospitals must become as efficient and as effective as possible. This conclusion sounds good and is certainly familiar, but it is incompatible with a key point from the previous chapter: Only one variable can be maximized or minimized in a system with limited resources. A goal of producing the highest possible quality of care at the lowest possible price simply "does not compute."

Therefore, health care's strategic decision makers must decide whether efficiency or effectiveness is the variable to be optimized by their organization. They must choose between: 1) being as efficient as possible for a fixed level of effectiveness, or 2) being as effective as possible for a fixed level of efficiency. Either option is defensible. However, for

two compelling reasons, the first choice—maximizing efficiency at a fixed level of effectiveness—is obvious when the
new marketplace imperatives are taken into account.

- Effectiveness defined in terms of quality should not be
a variable when consumers, who are spending more of
their own money on health care, can easily compare
the quality of competing providers. If consumers want
to know what they can reasonably expect from a hospital or medical group, quality should be a constraint
(i.e., services meet specific quality criteria because
they are produced according to standardized processes). Admittedly, studies have not yet demonstrated that
data on quality significantly influence consumers'
choice of providers, but the foundations for major
impact have only been set forth in the past year or
two. The era of informed consumers is too new for
definitive studies. However, the number of data-rich
resources for quality comparisons is proliferating, as is
the number of patients who now "have skin in the
game" with high-deductible health plans. Even a relatively low proportion of quality-informed consumers,
say one-third for argument' sake, would be enough to
justify fixing quality standards at a high level (see next
section) if—as can reasonably be expected—these are
the patients most likely to pay their bills. Accepting
variations in quality seems dangerous under the
emerging circumstances.

- Efficiency is the variable to maximize, once quality is
fixed. As indicated, the main reason for writing this
book comes from a conviction that hospitals must
learn to live with the level of real (i.e., inflation-

adjusted) revenues they currently receive. Payers and consumers are neither willing nor able to pay more money just to keep hospitals and doctors in business. Therefore, providers need to produce medical services as efficiently as possible. Operating costs must be cut because net revenues cannot be reliably increased. The difference between fixed revenues and declining costs—subject to the quality constraint, of course—is the only money that most providers can capture to make strategic investments in the personnel and technologies of 21st century health care.

Therefore, hospitals and medical groups need to become as efficient as possible in producing health services of prespecified quality. Efficiency is the variable. Quality-based, objectively defined effectiveness is the constraint. Both are imperative for the vast majority of providers.

Setting the Standard for Quality

This analysis implies the need for a major shift in thinking for provider organizations, from doing as well as possible with inconsistent and uncontrolled work processes (effectiveness with quality as a variable) to doing exactly what is promised with standardized work processes (effectiveness with quality as a fixed constraint). The strategic implications of this conclusion present a radical challenge to the status quo. Most providers must promptly confront serious shortcomings in their existing approaches to quality. In order to survive, they will need to adopt and enforce different production processes in organizations where tradition has not only allowed, but protected, an individual practitioner's freedom to practice medicine his or her own way.

This tradition substantially explains the wide variations in outcomes and unsustainable costs that are currently being addressed via reimbursement reform. However, pay for performance is at best an indirect mechanism for responding to the imperatives of the new medical marketplace, and the P4P thresholds are not much of a stretch from the traditional baseline. Providers can accomplish marginal improvement in compliance with quality indicators by making tactical changes. They are not compelled to make strategic changes, such as redesigning production processes or changing the personnel assigned to a task.

Hence, reimbursement reform is a "lite" approach to providing effective health care. It is incrementalism in the right direction, but it does not require any strategic changes that get to the crux of the quality and cost problems. Instead, providers need to intervene directly in the production of medical services. And they need to accomplish this clinical transformation on their own, sooner rather than later, because meaningful industry-wide solutions are unlikely to occur in the current political and economic environments.

Leading firms in other industries have solved their particular versions of this same quality problem. They made major changes in labor and capital allocation and reengineered production processes. They reexamined all aspects of doing business because the old ways of doing business weren't working any more. Many of the case studies presented in this book are about health care providers who borrowed successful production methods from transportation, banking, nuclear power, and manufacturing. They show that providers, acting on their own, can achieve world-class performance in terms of efficiency and effectiveness.

The Model for Defining Effectiveness

Transformation of the airline industry provides an excellent model for health care providers to follow. The effectiveness of commercial aviation was recognized as a serious problem in the last decades of the 20th century. Fatalities occurred at an unacceptable rate, so the industry engaged external experts to help isolate the causes of preventable crashes. (Not surprisingly, the ineffectiveness of health care is often described in terms of two or three 747s crashing every day—a scary and unflattering analogy that should shame the health care industry into action.) Careful studies showed that nearly all airline accidents were caused by human error.

Pilots with the most experience—ones with "all the right stuff"—frequently committed these fatal errors. The experts concluded that too much importance had been assigned to experience and not enough to the way pilots actually flew the planes. Airline crashes were almost completely eliminated when the carriers standardized flight procedures for all pilots. Simulators were used to assure consistency in training and performance. A culture of safety was created, with special mechanisms created to reward—not penalize—reporting of errors. All critical incidents were investigated and performance standards were updated as necessary to prevent them from happening again.

Commercial air crashes were almost completely eliminated by the beginning of the 21st century, thanks to the development *and enforcement* of performance standards, uniform training, team development, human factors engineering, and standardization of equipment. Paying a little bit more to pilots who followed the rules was not part of the solution. All pilots were expected to perform according to the new, standardized procedures. (Ironically, airlines discovered that their best pilots tended to be those hired with the FAA minimum number of flight hours. The least-experienced pilots were generally better at learning to fly safely by the book. Many of the most-experienced pilots had trouble conforming with standards because they had spent so many hours developing their own style of flying.)

Effectiveness in Health Care: Eliminating Avoidable Errors

Because lives are on the line in both industries, commercial aviation's compelling lesson for health care is to pursue the goal of absolute effectiveness: operating without avoidable errors. Hospitals and medical groups should adopt the tools of management engineering, performance improvement, and clinical transformation to ensure that any service is provided the right way, all the time. Once consistent and correct production techniques are established as the constraint, providers can then devote their efforts to maximizing efficiency.

Many readers will think the goal of eliminating avoidable errors is unreachable, so the chapters that follow explain viable approaches to efficiency and effectiveness—supported by successful case studies that show how health care can be delivered without avoidable errors. If skeptics remain, a simple question may suffice, "To save money, would you be willing to get your health care from a provider that publicly admits its care is not always as good as it could be?"

Most people wouldn't be any more willing to patronize this hospital or medical group than they would be to fly on an airline that admits it gets them (not just their luggage) to their destination most of the time. Hence, providers that accept the imperatives of efficiency and effectiveness must adopt the following goal for their mission statements: *Doing health care right all the time, as inexpensively as possible!* This statement should be in every strategic plan. The next chapter provides ideas regarding how to deliver on this promise.

| FOUR |

THE COMMON DENOMINATOR: INFORMATION TECHNOLOGY

Somewhere around seventh grade, school children learn about the common denominator as an essential key to solving quantitative problems. A multifactorial equation does not compute until every factor rests on the same numeric foundation. By analogy, a common denominator is fundamentally necessary for solving the problems of cost and quality in health care because processes for becoming efficient and effective are intensively data-driven. A staggering volume of information must be used to find the least-expensive way to provide health care free of unavoidable errors. The quantity of data related to the care of any patient is simultaneously growing at warp speed. All the information resources must be tied together in a common denominator—information technology (IT)—before meaningful progress can be made.

The information processing power required to produce medical services efficiently and effectively clearly transcends the capabilities of paper-based data systems. No other industry may be more data-driven than health care, but neither is any other significant U.S. industry less prepared to use its information productively. All health care stakeholders are stuck on a paper trail, and the trail does not lead to a better delivery system or a healthier nation. Health care simply cannot and will not reach its full potential until it is supported by a state-of-the-art infrastructure of IT. This obvious conclusion about the fundamental importance of IT leads to the remaining e-imperative embedded in this book's title.

e-Health: The Digital Transformation

The third e-imperative (in addition to efficiency and effectiveness) is e-health. The "e-" prefix is borrowed from the first letter of *electronic* and has been used to characterize corresponding technological advancement in a variety of domains (e.g., e-mail, e-commerce). Although e-health is used to encompass several different dimensions of health care, all the e- concepts reflect process automation made possible by computers and networks. Hence, by definition, e-health activities use the tools of the digital age to automate work that was previously done by people processing paper. Evolution of e-health will ultimately move providers close to a paperless environment. (Paper will not completely disappear any time soon. It will always have a few defensible uses in health care, such as reminder notes in a clinician's shirt pocket.)

E-health is used in this book as a synonym for *the digital transformation of health care*. The e-health imperative pushes providers to collect, store, process, analyze, and share information in digital formats. Paper records, from registration information through therapeutic and diagnostic data to billing forms, must be replaced with electronic databases that are processed by networked computers. The information of 21st-century health care must be simultaneously accessible to many people who have the need and the right to use it. The security of this information must be protected at the state of the art. Analytic systems must monitor the information and initiate interventions consistent with the imperatives of efficiency and effectiveness.

Fortunately, IT tools already exist to perform all these functions—as shown by many examples in this chapter. The adoption of e-health is imperative because old ways of sharing information waste limited resources in a marketplace where real revenues have peaked. Purchasers and payers are no longer willing or able to subsidize the inefficiency and ineffectiveness of paper-based medical care. They are beginning to expect hospitals, physicians, and other providers of health services to enter the world of 21st-century business practices. They are not imposing e-health, but they are expecting exchange relationships that can only be accomplished via digital transformation. Providers that do not convert to e-health will be lucky to be in business in the long run.

Two important components of e-health are often overlooked in general discussions of the digitization of medical services.

- First, digital transformation involves more than conversion from paper to electronic databases. It also encompasses the shift from analog to digital devices, such as the replacement of x-ray film with digital files in diagnostic imaging. A modern picture archiving and communications system (PACS) is an excellent example of an e-health tool that reduces production costs and standardizes quality.

- Second, digital transformation also involves more than information technology. Modern telecommunications systems are as important as computers and other digital devices. An excellent example of the fundamental importance of communications in e-health is telemedicine, a rapidly growing care delivery model that allows clinicians and patients to overcome long-standing barriers of place and time—efficiently and effectively.

Significantly, communications technology gets equal billing in the acronym used to describe e-health in Europe. Where Americans use IT (for information technology) in writings and discussions on the subject, Europeans use ICT (for information and communications technology). This book uses the IT acronym because it is written primarily for a U.S. audience. However, the term ICT recognizes that communications technology is an essential element in the big picture. State-of-the art information systems won't solve a lot of problems if they cannot communicate with each other. Connectivity and interactivity are as important as hardware and software.

Emulating Other Industries

Health care has a remarkably low level of automation for a personal services industry. For comparison, try to imagine a bank without an interactive network of automated teller machines (ATMs) that allow its customers to withdraw cash and make deposits, at any time of day in many convenient locations. An airline without online reservations, ticketing, and check-in is just as hard to picture in today's marketplace. A major retailer without an online store is equally unimaginable. Passbook savings accounts and paper tickets have effectively disappeared. Shopping from home is completely natural. Automation has been a win–win for sellers and buyers.

Any bank, airline, or national retailer that tried to force all its customers back into a line to conduct a transaction with a clerk would soon be out of business.

Yet the equivalents of tellers and paper tickets remain the norm in health care. Even at the end of 2007, the vast majority of health care delivery organizations did not have a complete electronic medical record (EMR), a longitudinally robust clinical data repository, a computerized practitioner order entry (CPOE) system, clinical decision support technology, or an electronic medication administration record (eMAR). Pharmacies, medical laboratories, and diagnostic imaging departments generally were automated with internal systems, but few of them could exchange information and interact with essential support functions inside the enterprise (e.g., scheduling, materials management, personnel). Some providers offered electronic portals where stakeholders could retrieve information, but few had anything close to the seamless systems consumers have come to expect from banks, airlines, retailers, and most other nonhealth businesses.

The road to full automation in hospitals and medical groups is going to be long and winding. According to the 18th Annual Health Care Information & Management Systems Society (HIMSS) Leadership Survey released in April 2007, only one-third of the respondents reported having a "fully operational" EMR in place. However, industry observers generally believe that the percentage of hospital organizations with "full" EMRs is actually quite small because the survey respondents are not representative of the industry as a whole. Providers that have already automated are presumably much more likely to participate in surveys about automation. Information technology professionals from HIMSS Analytics have been visiting hospitals and health systems across the country to determine for themselves which organizations have a "full" EMR system. Using an objective definition, they have regularly produced nationwide estimates in the single digits. Less than one hospital in ten has a fully functional EMR system. Most hospitals still need to automate their patient records.

Need for Growth in Information Systems

Regardless of who is counting and what they are counting, hospitals and medical groups have no choice but to install clinical information systems to reduce costs and meet quality standards. Labor costs, including the value of physicians' time, will continue rising due to limited supply. Hiring more labor is obviously a losing proposition in a marketplace where labor is getting more expensive and real revenues have quit rising. Providers simply cannot count on raising prices to cover higher costs of production. Consequently, productivity of the existing workforce must be improved. The next chapter provides an overview of proven techniques to improve performance in health care delivery organizations, but these tools for getting the most out of the workforce require extensive data analysis.

Increased investment in IT is the price to be paid for efficiency and effectiveness. Hiring more workers, even if they were available, would not solve the problems of cost and quality because these workers would need more and better information to do a better job. In terms of economic theory, health care is at the point where the marginal returns to IT are much higher than the marginal returns to labor. Increasing the supply of physicians and other health professionals will not produce anywhere near the benefits that can be obtained by increasing the information available to the workers already present. Information technology is a resource whose time has come.

Fortunately, health care leaders are coming to realize what must be done in the area of automation. A consensus on IT is developing across the industry and throughout the country. For example, nearly half the respondents in the 2007 HIMSS Leadership Survey assigned top priority to installing electronic medical records (EMR), computerized practitioner order entry (CPOE), clinical information systems, and bar-coded medication management systems. Reducing medical errors and promoting patient safety—in other words, responding to the effectiveness imperative—were identified as the most important reasons for assigning top priority to these specific IT applications.

These results need to be put into proper perspective. One-half of the respondents to one of the industry's most respected IT surveys would not have assigned top priority to quality-enhancing automation as recently as five years ago. Historically, respondents were much more interested in IT systems that generated bills, stored data, and managed materials. The only significant IT concerns in the clinical realm then were managing images (PACS) and diagnostic tests (radiology and laboratory information systems—RIS and LIS). Today's top survey concerns represent a rather remarkable shift in emphasis from systems that keep records to systems that enhance patient care. A large number of health care's IT professionals seem to recognize the efficiency and effectiveness imperatives.

Getting Started: First Steps with P4P

The need for system-wide action is obvious. Directors, senior executives, and clinical leaders who accept the cost and quality imperatives must move rapidly toward the automation of key processes. They must provide physicians, nurses, pharmacists, and other clinical specialists with the information to work efficiently and effectively. They must transparently provide purchasers, payers, and consumers with meaningful information to evaluate clinical performance and to compare prices. The leaders of nonprofit organizations must quantify their charitable contributions to the community, and the leaders of for-profit organizations must provide meaningful metrics to their investors. It's rapidly becoming a data–driven market. Robust IT is the only way for most providers to survive in it.

A federal agency, the Center for Medicare and Medicaid Services (CMS), is providing a positive glimpse into the future for all providers with its CMS/Premier Hospital Quality Incentive Demonstration Project (HQID). More than 260 hospitals nationwide are participating in this program that will help define the future relationship between efficiency, effectiveness, and payment. The provider organizations chosen to participate in this data-driven, policy-setting program are ramping up their information technologies to manage performance, measure outcomes, and support pricing. They are taking the pole position and will have a head start in the race to capture a self-sustaining share of a medical marketplace that no longer grows to subsidize high prices and low quality.

Although the policy outcomes of pay for performance (P4P) are far from certain, the advantages to the early adopters are obvious. They will set the benchmark standards. Under the current policy scenario, providers that fall short of the standards will get a lower reimbursement. To be fair, P4P is almost always described the other way around, in positive terms: providers that meet the standards will get a higher reimbursement. To be honest, the long-term outcome is most likely negative. Providers that do not meet the standards will not be reimbursed. Pay for performance is arguably much more radical than anything ever imagined by its creators: meet standards, or work for free. Investing in IT now may be essential to getting paid in the not-too-distant future because standards cannot be met without data.

Seeing the Forest, Leading the Way

Even organizations that do not face labor shortages will still need IT to be successful. (Imagine the outcome if banks had rejected ATMs and staked their future on hiring more tellers instead.) Being able to hire qualified employees at affordable wages does not exempt a provider from investing in systems that manage the growing volume of data that health care workers need to do their jobs. A hospital or medical group simply cannot hire enough labor to overcome a shortage of essential information. Uninformed workers will be unproductive workers, with serious negative consequences for efficiency and effectiveness. The cumbersome, inefficient, error-tolerant, paper-based systems of 20th-century health care and hospital operations must go away. The need for automation is obvious.

Organizations that are leading the way toward a responsible health system have made a firm commitment to efficiency, effectiveness, and e-transformation. For example, Tim Zoph, vice president and CIO at the 744-bed Northwestern Memorial Hospital in downtown Chicago, reports that his hospital completed well over 125 process improvement projects between 2004 and 2007. This (primarily) clinical activity was accompanied by a 57 percent reduction in potential avoidable harm. It was made possible by an ongoing investment of more than $100 million in clinical information systems. Zoph says the IT expenditures are worthwhile, especially when tied to optimization. "The value in these systems is not just in getting the initial adoption, but coupling implementation with process improvement and getting real change. We've trained 98 percent of our employees on GE's DMAIC methodology—define, measure, analyze, improve, and control. We embraced process improvement in parallel with installation of our electronic health record infrastructure. Having this IT infrastructure has given us the opportunity to improve care."

Similarly, New York's Memorial Sloan-Kettering Cancer Center decided to upgrade its enterprise IT system when operations were extended beyond the organization's 432-bed inpatient facility in Manhattan to Westchester County, New Jersey, and the Long Island suburbs in the late 1990s. Faced with a potential nightmare in medical records and clinical decision support resulting from the system's rapid expansion, Memorial Sloan-Kettering's leaders decided to forge ahead with a comprehensive automation plan. An electronic medical record (EMR) system and a picture archiving and communications system (PACS) were installed across the organization. "When we decided to broaden our base, we quickly realized that we couldn't have an efficient operation while moving paper records and x-ray film around the system," explains Patricia Skarulis, Memorial Sloan-Kettering's vice president and CIO. "So we digitized our paper records, installed our core EMR and PACS system, and got rid of all our films while we opened a new facility in Midtown."

Quality First

Once Skarulis and her colleagues at Memorial Sloan-Kettering had installed comprehensive clinical records systems, they had simultaneously created the capability to implement some exemplary process improvement programs (e.g., the forced-order system for VTE prophylaxis described in Chapter 5). The organization self-developed an extension of its commercial EMR system to give clinicians an overview of a patient's condition and care. The dashboard shows medication history and current medications, patient demographic data, and current physician notes. CMIO David Artz, MD, reports that this system is especially valuable because it provides current information when care is transferred from one resident to another. This IT add-on is a direct, proactive response to the Joint Commission on Accreditation of Health Care Organizations (JCAHO) recommendation that hospitals should carefully structure patient supervision handoffs, a common point of medical error.

An industry-wide consensus now clearly supports patient safety as sufficient justification for well-implemented IT projects. Medication management is a strong case in point. The closed-loop medication management system at the Brigham & Women's Hospital in Boston provides an excellent example of how IT can be customized to achieve desired effectiveness in patient safety. Clinicians at Brigham & Women's began their improvement process by conducting intensive studies of their previous processes for medication management. Careful analysis of the findings identified technology solutions that clinicians could use to prevent medication errors. Appropriate IT systems were then installed over a time frame that allowed adequate budgeting and preparation for successful implementation. As a result of this careful planning, the hospital's medication management system is widely seen as one of the best in the country.

Enhanced patient safety was also paramount when leaders of the 15-hospital, Milwaukee-based Ministry Health System decided to build a new hospital near Wausau. In collaboration with the Marshfield Clinic, one of the nation's most—respected comprehensive health systems, Ministry's leaders decided that the new facility would be all—digital from the beginning, with patient safety as the principal planning and operating objective. As a result, the 107-bed Saint Clare's Hospital opened in October 2005 as a virtual petri dish of patient safety improvement activity. Physicians and nurses were focused on becoming effective efficient in their day-to-day work. Thanks to CPOE, verbal orders—one of the most common causes of medical error—are virtually nonexistent. Larry Hegland, MD, the hospital's chief medical officer (CMO), notes, "We started talking about the safety-oriented, all-digital culture of this organization well before we opened. We planned to take advantage of the electronic system, and we encouraged people to report problems. As a result, we're often able to address problems in real time, while the patient is still here," he says.

Another common source of ineffective quality is documentation errors related to drug administration. Good Samaritan Hospital in Vincennes, Indiana, attacked this problem head-on by providing nurses with cart-mounted laptops linked to an IT system for bar-coded medications. The 267-bed hospital's chief information officer (CIO), Charles Christian, reports that nurses have fully integrated mobile computing into their clinical work flow. Now, 98 percent of all medications are being delivered to patients in bar-coded form, and documentation speed has improved considerably within a few months after full electronic tracking and monitoring of bar-coded medication administration at the bedside.

Results at 319-bed United Hospital Center in Clarksburg, West Virginia, also confirm the critical importance of IT systems to reducing human error in health care delivery. The hospital's CIO, Edmund Collins, reports, "With a mobile clinical system that integrates bedside documentation with bar-coded drug administration, we have reduced medication errors around 75 percent." The wireless network behind the hospital's system allows clinicians to use a variety of interface devices consistent with different work flows.

Obvious progress is being made across the industry. Information technology investments are yielding desired returns in a broad range of operational areas. Given the top priority put on quality—proudly and proactively imposing the constraint of doing health care right, all the time—all hospitals can soon have success stories like those presented in this section. Looking 10 years ahead, hospital leaders and industry observers will, hopefully, look back on the quality of care with a mix of horror and relief—horror at the poor overall quality of the past (our present) and relief that care in their day (our future) sets the standard for other countries to follow. Digital transformation of the delivery of medical services now is the only viable path to a future of better care for everyone.

Value of IT Confirmed

One sign of progress toward world-class health care in the United States is an emerging consensus on how IT investments should be sequenced. Chief information officers (CIOs) of industry-leading hospitals and health systems not only agree on the focus of their IT budgets (i.e., automated systems that manage work flow to achieve targeted performance goals), but also on the overall thrust of IT needs to support the enterprise's desired strategic direction. Chief information officers are becoming proactively involved in actions to meet system-wide goals. The national leaders are managing and measuring IT resources to promote efficiency and effectiveness for the enterprise, not for the IT department. Trustees, senior executives, and clinical leaders should not only expect this global focus from their IT leaders, but also welcome them into full membership of the strategic team.

The point is well made by Stephanie Reel, vice president and CIO of the Johns Hopkins Health System, Baltimore, Maryland. "When I think about the trends in health care, I think about rising costs, uneven quality, labor shortages, increasing demand, information overload, and other challenges that are not the traditional concerns of IT. Frankly, we CIOs are starting to think first about global interdependencies and then about technology." She concludes, "We think about our role in mitigating those system-wide risks by reducing waste, by facilitating collaboration, by providing evidence of best practices, and by finding more sustainable uses of health care resources."

Sustainability is a concept that also resonates with David Muntz, senior vice president of information services and CIO at the Baylor Health Care System in Dallas. "The true value of IT is not that you can do new things exceedingly well, but that IT allows you to achieve sustainability in the things you've already got while you're trying to achieve new things. IT departments have done amazing things in terms of improving quality, but we haven't always been focused on sustainability." Muntz gives the example of clinical decision support tools that can help clinicians achieve immediate improvements in quality of clinical care, but he says that a newly installed system can become static over time. Information technology professionals need to understand that clinicians' work lives are changing by the day. A system that is state of the art when installed can quickly become outdated if not managed as a dynamic support service.

"Computers are relentless in the pursuit of consistency," he notes. Information technology resources must be managed to adapt to the changes because new things are always being demanded of health systems.

James Mormann, vice president of the Des Moines-based Iowa Health System with 2,300 beds in eleven hospitals, is sensitive to the same challenge. "IT can provide great value because it is logically consistent over time. After all, computers process nothing but zeros and ones. How computers work is not going to change any time soon, but computer applications will be changing all the time." Consequently, Mormann sees IT as a facilitator, not a generator, of change. "If a provider is trying to become efficient and effective—which, in my mind, are fancy words for process change—IT will have problems unless it is a foundation of process change," he says. "IT is an extremely powerful facilitator when it is an integral part of standardizing processes. Neither process change nor IT are sufficient on their own; they must work hand in hand."

Teamwork + Work Flow = Process Improvement

In the final analysis, these IT success stories result from close collaboration. All stakeholders are involved for the resulting improvement of the enterprise—that is, for making their particular contributions to the common goals of reducing costs and producing services of defined quality. Although health care lags far behind other industries in responding to serious economic threats with IT, ample evidence suggests that health care has many exemplary IT leaders who approach the future as strategic, "big picture" thinkers. In addition, this chapter's first-hand reports, supported by hundreds of articles in the trade press and academic journals, clearly demonstrate that IT is an essential tool for solving health care's cost and quality problems. Trustees and chief executives must see digital transformation as an essential part of the solution and must have IT leaders who work synergistically throughout the enterprise.

Manual processes cannot provide the needed synergy at the bottom line. They become inefficient and ineffective as medical care becomes more complex. The requirements for clinical competence in the 21st century indisputably exceed the capacities of clinicians working from paper records. Of course, a few caregivers will think they can do "just fine" without IT. Even if they do claim perfect recall and flawless intuition, their knowledge does not extend to other members of the team, in all times and places when it might be needed. Today's health care is a team activity because no individual can possess all the knowledge and skills to meet a patient's needs "24-7." Everyone on the team needs access to a common information resource that supports a proven system of care.

To conclude by merging two key points of this chapter, IT solutions need to support the work flow requirements of a team of caregivers. And providers and vendors need to work together to create IT tools that channel all workers' efforts in a predetermined direction, minimizing the costs of producing medical services of predetermined quality. Stephen Davidson, MD, chairman of the Department of Emergency Medicine at Maimonides Medical Center in Brooklyn, New York, puts it best, saying, "The issue is supporting work flow. And that's what so many IT vendors keep missing. Clinicians want tools that support work flow."

Following Chapter 5, which relates 12 case studies from pioneering provider organizations across the United States,

Chapter 6 provides an executive-level overview of the tools of process improvement. Leaders should make sure that their organizations are using these tools to identify wasted resources and redirect them to productive uses through intelligent work flow design.

| FIVE |

BECOMING EFFICIENT AND EFFECTIVE: CASE STUDIES

Case studies show how to put economic theory into successful practice, and fortunately, there is no dearth of health systems, hospitals, and medical groups that have become efficient and effective by making the necessary strategic changes over the past few years. The case studies in this chapter demonstrate that providers can set and meet top quality standards *and* cut operating costs in the process.

In these studies, efficiency and effectiveness almost always went hand in hand. Projects designed to meet objectives in one domain tended to produce gains in the other, too. This "two for the price of one" discovery changed our original plans for separate groupings of case studies on efficiency and effectiveness. In fact, the two economic objectives become so intertwined that there is no sensible way to separate them into two chapters as originally planned.

Instead, this single long chapter provides a rich collection of success stories from a wide range of provider organizations, including hospitals, medical groups, and integrated health systems. These case studies should inspire leaders who understand the imperatives but need encouragement and examples to start doing what needs to be done. The reports provide practical guides for action by showing how a small selection of similar organizations has improved its clinical and economic performance. Here, in no particular order, are a dozen success stories that illustrate the possibilities for efficiency and effectiveness in health care. (Regrettably, several equally meritorious success stories needed to be excluded to keep this chapter from becoming too long.)

Medication Management: Brigham & Women's Hospital

Medication management is one of the most complex problems in health care. It encompasses many organizational functions and involves personnel from an array of departments. No wonder, then, that the vast majority of patient safety studies identify medication management as the most common area for errors in hospital-based care. Surveys have found that the average U.S. health care consumer, patient, or family member knows someone who personally experienced a medication error. In April, 2007, the Agency for Healthcare Research and Quality (AHRQ) reported that adverse drug events (ADE) were found in 3.1 percent of all hospital stays.

Medication errors are not only devastating in terms of mortality; they are also costly to the health care system. Numerous studies have shown that the average ADE adds thousands of dollars to the cost of caring for the unlucky patient. The cumulative economic cost can be millions of dollars per year in a large hospital. Given the tremendous costs and potential harm to patients, many outside observers have expressed dismay that the problem has not been eliminated. Insiders respond by noting the complexity of the process and the need for a robust IT infrastructure, one that encompasses electronic medical records (EMR), computerized practitioner order entry (CPOE), electronic medication administration records (eMAR), and pharmacy information systems in order to prevent human errors. Only a handful of U.S. hospitals have put the whole package together, saving lives and money. One of the leaders in this area is Brigham & Women's Hospital, a large academic medical center and part of the Partners Health system in the Boston area.

Like the vast majority of American hospitals, Brigham & Women's had a traditional 24-hour medication administration system, one in which the hospital's pharmacy prepared unit doses that were transported to the floors and stored in drug cabinets on nursing units. Brigham's pharmacists spent most of their time filling individual medication orders or supervising the work of pharmacy technicians. Frustrated nurses spent many hours doing work-arounds in order to obtain medications in a timely manner for their patients. William Churchill, MS, the hospital's executive director of pharmacy services, recalls what nurses used to tell him about the old system, "You call it unit-dose; we call it floor stock, sorted by patient." Because nurses often did not know when medications were due to be delivered or to be given to the patients, they created multiple "stashes" of medications tucked away in drawers on patient floors. Not surprisingly, this haphazard system—typical in hospitals throughout the country—led to numerous errors. Patients could receive the wrong medications, the wrong doses, or even the right medications at the wrong time.

Churchill and other clinician leaders convened attending physicians, residents, nurse managers, floor nurses, pharmacists, pharmacy techs, and other personnel in 2000 and engaged them in in-depth discussions about all the actual process for medication management at the hospital. They uncovered the bottlenecks and workarounds, and they all worked together to design an innovative closed-loop medication-management process built on a foundation of EMR, CPOE, pharmacy automation, and eMAR.

Multidisciplinary teams were assigned to create specifications for the pharmacy system, to design a two-dimensional bar code and a bar code repackaging center (because less than one-third of all medications had bar codes upon delivery to the hospital), to select robotics for the pharmacy, and to accomplish other key tasks. Meanwhile, the hospital's information services (IS) development team worked closely with the hospital's clinicians over nine months to write and design the new system and to write the code. Numerous innovations were built into the system, including a comprehensive medication-tracking system that used the hospital's two-dimensional bar code system. Another innovation was the implementation of a smart infusion pump system from a leading vendor.

Medication safety was improved by many procedural innovations, such as a process change involving how pharmacy orders flowed through the hospital. "Under the old system, nursing and pharmacy got medication orders independently," Churchill notes. "In the old, paper-based MAR system, the nurse—often frustrated by the slow delivery of medications—would see the order from the physician before the pharmacy did and would often get a medication ordered for a different patient or from a stash, even though the dose might be different." The new system is designed to prevent a nurse from acting on a physician order until pharmacy has reviewed that order. It has also optimized efficiency of order processing by assigning one of three levels of timeliness to the order, clustering medication orders into prioritization cues for the pharmacists, and streamlining prescription filling. Orders are now filled in a highly efficient manner, averting the former need for nurse workarounds. Indeed, nurses and pharmacists are now working out of a single, integrated eMAR system with a bidirectional interface.

Because of the vast improvement over the old order-filling system, pharmacists have been freed from many previous functions. Pharmacists now spend most of their workdays doing multidisciplinary rounds with the other clinicians and analyzing patients' medications. Today, pharmacists might request a change of dose or frequency of administration, or they might intervene to discontinue use of a particular medication as warranted by an individual patient's situation. In addition, pharmacists are using wireless laptops on patient floors while doing their rounds with other clinicians. In short, pharmacists at Brigham & Women's now focus much more on patient care and much less on dispensing. As a result of all these performance improvements, pharmacists made nearly 12,000 clinical interventions on physician medication orders in 2006. In addition, the two-dimensional bar code-based system has led to 7,000 "hard stops" per month, preventing administration errors. These "catches" represent 2 percent of all medications administered, with up to 80 percent of the "hard stops" for the wrong drug, Churchill notes.

The implications of these accomplishments are quite impressive, even astonishing. The average patient at Brigham & Women's Hospital is taking 19 medications, Churchill notes. The average nurse is caring for four to five patients at

a time on one shift and following up to 600 different medication administrations (because each medicine is generally
administered multiple times throughout the shift). Even a one
percent error rate on 600 dosages represents six medication
errors per nurse per day. Given that his organization administers six million medication doses every year and that a 20
percent medication administration error rate is the rule of
thumb in the industry, Churchill notes that a large academic
medical center could be experiencing as many as one million
medication errors a year. Brigham & Women's has obviously
saved a lot of money and lives by reengineering its medication administration system.

The final links between the hospital's eMAR and
CPOE systems were being put into place as this book went
to press. Looking at the vast project, Michael Gustafson, MD,
Brigham's vice president for clinical excellence, says that,
"When you think about medication safety, you have to think
about the complete electronic closed-loop medication
administration system, from the time the physician orders the
medication to when the nurse administers the medication to
the patient." To enhance efficiency and effectiveness, process
changes must be made and coordinated across the entire system. It also takes some money. Gustafson says that Brigham &
Women's has spent roughly $10 million on all its medication-
related innovations. Still, he says, the hospital sees a long-term
return on its investment, measured in terms of lower costs
and standardized quality, "Success was achieved largely by
standardizing clinical practice at the level of the nurse, the
physician, and the pharmacist, and by reducing unnecessary
variation," Gustafson notes. The success at Brigham &
Women's shows the importance of formal programs to eliminate unnecessary variation.

Supply Chain Management: Virginia Commonwealth University Health System

Virginia Commonwealth University Health System (VCUHS) in Richmond, Virginia, is an integrated health system anchored by the 779-bed VCU Medical Center (VCUMC). Four years ago, its leaders made a commitment to manage supply chain costs aggressively. Like other academic medical centers, VCUMC derives a significant portion of its revenues from cardiac surgery, angioplasty, cardiac catheterization, and other "big-ticket" invasive procedures. With the rapidly rising cost of supplies for those procedures, VCUHS was experiencing severe impact at the bottom line.

The management team at VCUHS decided to create a philosophy and approach to supply costs that would set it apart from its counterparts. "Developing a comprehensive mindset was crucial to the success of VCUHS's attack on supply costs," says John F. Duval, the medical center's CEO. "We have a responsibility to be good stewards with our resources, so defining a rational and clinically appropriate approach to supply spending is part of our job." To that end, he initiated an enterprise-wide review of supply costs through the organization's hospital alliance, University HealthSystem Consortium (UHC), based in Oak Brook, Illinois.

Duval put Timothy Wildt, director of resource management, in charge of day-to-day management of supply costs. Through intensive data mining, Wildt helped teams of clinicians and support staff uncover broad areas of opportunity for savings. The bottom line? VCUHS's comprehensive approach has yielded an annual savings of nearly $3 million on total spending of $18 million to $20 million. Behind these marquee numbers are a $1 million cost reduction in electrophysiology, where the health system's annual spending on pacemakers and defibrillators is about $7 million, and $350,000 savings on cardiac stents, where annual costs have averaged around $2 million.

How has VCUHS achieved this impressive improvement in efficiency? The key has been a clever combination of data management, strategy, culture change, and communication. In every area, executives have created ongoing dialogues with key physicians in the specialty area involved and have obtained their permission to allow buyers to challenge vendors on pricing, with the understanding that some narrowing of brand choice would inevitably occur. Rigorous data mining around utilization and cost patterns has been essential to this effort, along with monthly dissemination of resulting reports to key clinician leaders.

For example, Wildt performed comprehensive market research on the cost of drug-eluting stents to all the hospitals in the region. He analyzed costs by type and vendor and presented the results to the hospital's chair of cardiology. With the cardiology chair's consent, Wildt then went back to the three stent vendors in the regional market and got the second-place vendor to reduce its prices to VCUHS. Then, through a volume shift to that vendor, the volume leader reduced its prices to VCUHS as well.

The key takeaway here, Wildt says, is that a team must have and follow a strategy of thorough data mining and data analysis, beginning with a corporate culture that supports the necessary administrator–physician dialogue. Meanwhile, Wildt and members of his team are already looking to the future. They are developing a comprehensive initiative to understand the relationship between supply costs and clinical outcomes. This extension of VCUHS's already successful program offers even more opportunities for finding the least-expensive way (efficiency) to meet top-level quality standards (effectiveness).

Central-Line Infection Reduction: Allegheny General and Virginia Mason

The old adage about hospitals as dangerous places to recover could not be more apt than in the case of central-line infections, a potentially life-threatening result of placing central venous catheters in patients' major veins (e.g., neck, chest, groin) for cardiovascular monitoring, viable administration of intravenous drugs and fluids, etc. The numbers are staggering. An estimated 250,000 cases of central-line bloodstream infections (BSIs) occur in U.S. hospitals every year, with a resulting mortality rate as high as 25 percent for each infection, according to federal statistics. The additional cost to the health care system has been estimated as high as $56,000 per case. The resulting annual cost of caring for patients with central-line-associated BSIs is potentially $2.3 billion annually. Eliminating this problem would liberate a tidy sum for reallocation to other needs in provider organizations.

The problem of central-line-associated infections encompasses quality, patient safety, outcomes, and cost. Paradoxically, experts note that central-line infection prevention is not an inherently complex problem from a clinical standpoint. Rather, the challenge is process change. A number of pioneering hospitals nationwide have used this awareness to achieve dramatic reductions in central-line bloodstream infections. Two programs that stand out are at Allegheny General

Hospital in Pittsburgh and Virginia Mason Medical Center in Seattle.

In Pittsburgh, Allegheny General Hospital has been one of the lead hospitals participating in the BSI-reduction initiative of the Pittsburgh Regional Healthcare Initiative (PRHI). The PRHI's BSI reduction initiative took place between 2001 and 2005 and produced dramatic results: BSI rates among ICU patients declined 68 percent, from 4.31 to 1.35 per 1,000 central-line days. Allegheny General has done especially well among participating hospitals. Beginning in 2003, clinician leaders there introduced a standardized central-line insertion process in the hospital's coronary care unit. Jerome Granato, MD, medical director of Allegheny's coronary care unit, explains, "I call central-line insertion the 'caboose' of ICU procedures. It is frequently performed by residents, the least-trained individuals on the unit. Those residents historically have been trained by word of mouth, according to the old 'see one, do one, teach one' approach." That process is inherently flawed, he says. Just by standardizing the simplest of aspects of insertion—dressing wounds in the same way, using the same cleansing solution (chlorhexidine solution) to scrub the wound, and using impregnated patches on the wound—he and his colleagues "took a very big bite out of the infection rate."

Granato and his colleagues began doing real-time review of infections, consciously modeling their work on Toyota Production System (TPS) principles. Instead of waiting for a retrospective quarterly review of any occurrence, they reviewed any incident the very next day to determine its cause. That single decision reduced infections dramatically. Unfortunately, BSIs began to rise again several months later because of the regular turnover of residents. This observation led Granato and his colleagues to institute enduring, systemic changes. Dr. Granato himself authored a comprehensive and standardized training program in 2005, one required for all residents and nurses inserting central-line catheters. Intensive care unit caregivers must pass a written test and demonstrate technical mastery on a mannequin. The hospital has, at press date, gone 15 consecutive months in its coronary care unit without a single infection following implementation of the training program. In 2003, that unit had seen 49 BSIs in 35 patients (because some became infected twice). In 2006, that number was zero—a perfect example of effectiveness!

Clinicians at Seattle's Virginia Mason Medical Center (VMMC) have had a similar experience with central-line infection improvement. Clinician leaders there spent some time analyzing the causes of BSIs, says Cathie Furman, RN, MHA, the teaching hospital's senior vice president for quality and compliance. As at Allegheny, the clinician leaders at Virginia Mason had to overcome a basic problem, the lack of a standardized, systematized way to insert central lines.

Now, reports Charleen Tachibana, RN, Virginia Mason's senior vice president and chief nursing officer, a protocol is in place and is strictly followed. The clinician who inserts a central-line catheter must fully "gown up" (i.e., don gown, mask, and gloves, as if for surgery); the patient must be covered with sterile drapes, also as in an operating room. And a very specific clinical protocol defines which vessels are acceptable for insertion. The patient must also be evaluated every day to determine whether or not the line is still needed.

Finally, the clinician is required to perform a specific test to ensure that the line is being inserted into the correct vessel. The procedure is built into the electronic record, requiring nurses to verify necessity each day as a part of the clinical documentation process. Only 10 out of the hospital's 600 nurses are permitted to insert a peripherally inserted central line. As a result of the rigorous systematization of these processes, the central-line-associated BSI rate per 1,000 device days at Virginia Mason has declined dramatically in the hospital's critical care units, from 7.73 in 2002 to 2.81 in 2006.

Bed Management: Genesys Health System

As more hospitals move toward full-capacity utilization, their leaders are coming to realize that a bed-management program is needed to cut costs and maintain quality. Adding bed capacity through construction is not necessarily the economically sensible solution to the problem. The economic theory of efficiency suggests that getting better utilization of existing beds should always be explored first and will generally be the better approach. Until recently, few hospitals had maximized efficiency in this area; inefficient use of existing beds was the norm. But many hospitals are moving quickly now to improve bed management, especially when they cannot reasonably expect increases in real income to cover the costs of new construction.

Genesys Health System in Flint, Michigan, is a progressive organization that has focused on getting optimal use of existing beds. JoAnne Herman, vice president of clinical programs, reports that Genesys' main facility, Genesys Regional Medical Center at Health Park, has been running at about 85 percent capacity for some time. Executives at Genesys carefully considered the cost of "building out" new beds and concluded that improving efficiency of existing beds was clearly the better choice. (Economists generally define 85 percent utilization as full capacity. Moving from 85 percent to 100 percent utilization almost always increases costs, reduces quality, demoralizes employees, and annoys customers.)

Genesys Regional Medical Center had a standalone bed-management system in place, but only for the housekeeping department. With the goal of optimizing patient flow throughout the hospital's patient-care process, Herman and her colleagues worked in teams to analyze the challenge and to break it into discrete components. They analyzed all identifiable options, and agreed that the focus should be on quickly placing patients in medical/surgical beds from the emergency department, the operating room, or from other providers' facilities. The teams analyzed different care units (ICU, telemetry, labor and delivery beds) and looked at multiple measures, including patient-diversion rates, occupancy levels, lengths of stay, and the mechanics of bed management.

They designed a bed-management program that went live in mid 2006. Implementation is still being completed as this book goes to press, but Herman says she and her colleagues can already see clear improvement in efficiency. Large amounts of paper forms have been eliminated, patient-management processes have been nicely streamlined, and the process' method of systematization is being adopted for other aspects of inpatient operations. Even though final economic results are pending, all are pleased with the decision to focus on getting better use of existing beds rather than building new ones.

Medical Group Process Optimization: Crystal Run Health Care

Gregory Spencer, MD, a leader at Crystal Run Health Care, LLP, a large medical group in Middleton, New York, likes to tell a car purchasing story to explain his organization's core philosophy. "Several years ago," says Spencer (an internist and the group's chief medical information officer), "just at the time we were beginning to open up a new building for the practice, my managing partner (Hal Teitelbaum, MD) set out to buy a Hummer. It was a snowy night in December, and when he approached the door of the dealership, it had just closed. But they reopened just for him. Not only did he have a quality experience, but they assigned him a personal services coordinator to ensure that he would continue to have a good experience on the path towards receiving the new vehicle from the manufacturer. Dr. Teitelbaum came back to our group and said, 'Why can't we do that in health care? It's customer service, pure and simple.'" That idea—that Crystal Run Medical Group should constantly improve the patient experience at all levels, including customer service, clinical quality, and efficiency—has animated the practice-management efforts of Spencer and his colleagues ever since.

"I frequently tell our staff that the Golden Rule applies in everything we do, whether in interacting with physicians, employees, or anyone else. We will do unto others as we would do unto our families," says Teitelbaum. "And that means hiring the best people we possibly can. And we take a systematic approach to quality and safety, avoiding errors, and constantly improving the patient experience."

Not surprisingly, with that core philosophy driving the Crystal Run physicians, their group's growth has been exponential since 1996, when the group was an oncology practice with only a dozen physicians. Now, the organization's 125+ clinicians care for patients from seven locations across the mid-Hudson Valley and lower Catskill regions of New York State. The staff encompasses more than 20 specialties, from primary care to specialties such as surgery, urology, orthopedics, and oncology.

An organizational culture of entrepreneurial spirit and customer service underlies everything that goes on at Crystal Run, Teitelbaum and Spencer report. It has led directly to several important initiatives for ever-better care (effectiveness) and cost management (efficiency). First, the group has implemented an innovative Care Management Program (CMP), which gives physicians access to data at the point of care and maximizes compliance with routine wellness and health check-related protocols (e.g., ensuring that patients are informed when due for diagnostic tests). The group's EMR prompts clinicians to check wellness screenings, immunizations, and other important clinical data sets to maximize the efficiency of each office visit.

Patients are urged to enroll in the Care Management Program, and they are assigned an individual nurse who reviews their medical record to assess risk factors and coordinate health maintenance or disease-management activities. The CMP has also helped Crystal Run physicians achieve high levels of compliance with screening guidelines recommended by the National Committee for Quality Assurance (NCQA). For example, Crystal Run's level of prostate-specific antigen (PSA) screening compliance is over 90 percent, and compliance with mammography screening is 80 percent every year. Crystal Run's top-level performance is a direct result of its leadership's focus on process improvement to eliminate waste and meet quality standards.

Success in performance improvement reinforces another key component of Crystal Run's strategic orientation—participation in the Physician Office Link component of the NCQA's Bridges to Excellence program. Health plans around the country employ NCQA standards to reward physician groups for documented implementation of specific processes to reduce errors and increase quality. Crystal Run participates with several local health plans in this program. The group's leaders estimate that the Care Manager Program alone generates more than $150,000 annually in additional income through participation in such programs. Finally, the group's EMR provides an essential foundation for all its programs to be efficient and effective. It streamlines work flow, maximizes productivity, and provides robust business intelligence data for growth and market penetration. All this work has resulted, not only in healthier patients, but in a well-deserved and healthier bottom line for the group as well.

Essentially, the economic goal is doing what's right for patients and being rewarded for it. "We try to control our own destiny and use all the data and tools that are available, not just within the health care industry, but within the business world in general, to take better care of patients and maintain the financial viability of our enterprise," Dr. Spencer notes. "Crystal Run physicians are continually seeking additional opportunities to become more efficient and more effective and to enhance the patient experience." The group's leaders are considering a text-messaging service for patient appointment reminders, lab results, and other routine communications. "The service will only be selected for implementation if it fits within the practice's philosophy of enhanced service to the patient," Spencer adds.

Dr. Teitelbaum, whose energy and core philosophy have energized this exemplary group culture, recognizes that he and his colleagues have a vastly different mindset from most other physicians in private practice. "Physicians are good at whining and talking about the 'good old days,'" he says. "The truth is, there never really were good old days! If we're going to be happy for the remaining years of our practice, we have to get back to basics and respond to what customers want. I used to think entrepreneurialism was a dirty word in health care, but I ultimately came to realize that it was actually necessary. Health care would never improve unless people set their minds to improving things and took the initiative."

Nurse Efficiency Transformation: Virginia Mason Medical Center

For decades now, many hospitals have assigned their medical/surgical floor nurses to individual patients. It's a tradition based on the theory that better care and efficiency would result. However, in response to growing economic and consumer pressures, some hospitals have analyzed this practice model, come to a different conclusion, and redirected their nurse staffing as a result. One leader among those provider organizations with a new perspective is Virginia Mason Medical Center (VMMC) in Seattle, which has transitioned to a purely geographically based nurse assignment system (i.e., nurses are no longer assigned to specific patients). How did Virginia Mason's nursing leadership come to make this important change? Clinician leaders there carefully studied patient-based and acuity-based nurse assignment models and made strategic changes based on what they learned. They discovered that their nurses were spending only 36 percent of their workday on patient care—a figure that closely matches averages reported in many studies conducted throughout the country.

In terms of the workaday experience of the individual floor nurses, assigning nurses to specific individual patients turned out to be detrimental to their efficiency, according to

Charleen Tachibana, RN, Virginia Mason's senior vice president and chief nursing officer. In fact, she says, "We were losing efficiency and effectiveness by attempting to balance patient acuity levels through staffing."

Given their comprehensive adoption of the Toyota Production System (TPS), Virginia Mason's leaders decided to institute a series of rapid process improvement workshops. The goal was to learn how to move their nurses to where the patients were. In 2006, they tried the new concepts on a "test" floor where they implemented a new system of enhanced visual signaling which included the creation of signage (in the form of colored flags outside rooms) to indicate which patients were at increased risk for falls, which rooms had clean beds ready to accept new patients, and so on. They also reengineered the supply system in order to bring supplies closer to nurses' reach, and they reworked the nursing documentation process by instituting real-time documentation. Instead of nurses gathering in the conference room on each floor at the end of every shift to document care in the hospital's EMR, they were provided with computers on carts (known in the industry as "computers on wheels," or "COWS") and asked to document in real time at the bedside.

Further, Tachibana reports, "We began looking at everything that took the nurse out of the patient room; we documented and tracked everything." One resulting change was reengineering the transmission of verbal end-of-shift reports, moving those reports from the nurses' station. Nurses were subsequently required to report to each other verbally in front of patients, in the patients' rooms. Any psychosocial or other delicate issues are still handled away from any patient's hearing, but most patients, and often their families, can now hear first hand what nurses have to say to each other and can express wishes and preferences. They can see how clinicians discuss patient care issues, which means greater transparency has been introduced into the process as requested by a growing number of purchasers, payers, policy makers, and patients.

The results of all these changes have been dramatic. Nurses' time spent on direct patient care has been raised from 36 percent to 90 percent of their time—a very efficient outcome, given the shortage of nurses and the resulting increase in their cost to a hospital. This work has been typical of the many innovations taking place at VMMC, says Christina Saint Martin, the hospital's vice president for governance and administration. "We are continuously looking at how well the system [of patient care delivery and hospital operations] flows, at calculating the percentage of value-added versus non-value-added time in our processes, at creating a "pull system," in which the customers—internal or external—get what they want when they need it, and finally, at eliminating defects throughout the system."

Not surprisingly, the process changes have led to significant benefits for everyone. Efficiency and cost effectiveness have improved because the hospital has not needed to hire additional nurses to meet patient-care volume increases. Meanwhile, on the quality front, patients' clinical problems have been recognized and addressed earlier. Patient mortality has dropped. Code alerts—where patients go into cardiac arrest while in the hospital—have declined. Finally, having nurses report verbally to each other in front of patients at shift changes has led to greater redundancy in surveillance over problem areas such as medication administration. As this case study demonstrates, high-level performance improvement work inevitably encompasses both efficiency and effectiveness and improves both.

Geisinger Health System: ProvenCare Program

Geisinger Health System (GHS) provides care to 2.5 million people in 40 counties across northeastern and central Pennsylvania from its base in Danville. Geisinger Health System took a surprising and unprecedented step in February 2006, when it launched the ProvenCare program. For the first time in the history of the health care industry, a hospital-based organization set a guaranteed, publicly announced price on a major surgical procedure (coronary artery bypass graft, or CABG), and tied that transparent pricing initiative to its own internally developed, quality optimization program. Geisinger's leaders had not only committed to a set of CABG prices that purchasers and payers could bank on, they also publicly committed to continuous clinical-quality improvement activities that would create the efficiencies required to support the guaranteed pricing strategy.

Within the first year of the program's operation (through February 2007), length of stay for CABG decreased by 16 percent, and clinical outcomes improved dramatically. In-hospital mortality for bypass surgery dropped from 1.5 percent to 0 percent, ICU readmission dropped 69 percent (from 2.9 percent to 0.9 percent), pulmonary complications dropped from 7.3 percent to 2.6 percent, and readmission within 30 days dropped from 6.6 percent to 5.1 percent. Indeed, Ronald Paulus, MD, the health system's chief technology & innovation officer, says, "The program has either met or exceeded our high initial expectations." He adds, "We learned how to overcome one of the main gaps in improving care, namely being able to systematically bridge the gap between what theoretically should be done and what can actually be done."

The program emerged from a board of directors' mandate to focus on innovation as a strategic priority for the organization. It evolved over a period of months in 2005 and 2006, as several working groups were formed to focus on best practices and processes for CABG. Financial workgroups were formed, too, along with a steering committee established to supervise the overall process. Clinicians on the best-practices workgroup labored to translate evidence-based guidelines from respected sources such as the American College of Cardiology and the American Heart Association into 41 discrete procedural steps that would provide measurement and benchmark foundations for the program. The process of care workgroup analyzed clinical work flow across all dimensions of bypass surgery. The financial workgroup, which included the CFOs from the system's hospitals where CABGs were performed, developed financial scenarios and a pricing plan. Under the final program, Geisinger charges a flat fee for CABG surgery, plus half the historical cost of related care for the next 90 days. The health system absorbs any extra cost related to extended length of stay or readmission. The price point comes out to between $25,000 and $30,000 per surgery in 2007.

An absolute key to physician buy-in was an opt-out option, Paulus says. That plan allows a physician to opt out of any of the 41 procedural steps each time he or she performs CABG surgery, but it requires the doctor to explain why. In practice, very few have chosen to opt out of any of the recommended steps. Providing the option has created essential physician buy-in, Dr. Paulus notes. Paulus reports that "The cardiac team is proud, and rightfully so, of what they've accomplished in developing ProvenCare CABG. The fear factor has gone down somewhat over time."

What's more, he says, members of the team realize that "This is a continuous process of improvement. They are already revisiting the evidence base, based on some new studies that have come out, and they continue to tinker with the specific steps in the process in order to make it even better."

Most of all, Paulus credits the Geisinger Health System's clinical and organizational culture with the success of the ProvenCare program. From the organization's physician CEO, Glenn Steele, MD and its highly committed board to its clinicians and staff, he says that Geisinger has the right kind of culture to foster this type of world-class innovation. He adds that this remarkable example of efficiency and effectiveness could not have been achieved without the facilitation of enterprise-wide clinical information systems, including the organization's EMR.

Of course, the Geisinger team isn't about to stop at its success with CABG. At press time, successful pilot programs had been launched for hip replacement and for cataract surgery, with the same operating principles (guaranteed price, evidence-based step-by-step protocols, multidisciplinary team-based development). What's more, Eastern Pennsylvania's employer-purchasers have expressed a strong interest in a broader menu of guaranteed-price procedures. For Paulus and his colleagues, such developments are to be expected as the health care system moves toward even greater consumer centrism. Geisinger Health System certainly is determined to remain at the head of the pack as health care responds to significant changes in the marketplace. It clearly understands the imperatives and knows how to respond to them.

ED and PICC:
New York-Presbyterian

Hospital leaders across the country are acutely aware of the need to become efficient in their emergency departments (ED). Not only are EDs extremely expensive to operate, but they also affect costs throughout the entire facility. At New York-Presbyterian Hospital (NYP) in New York City, executives and clinicians have been intensively involved in performance improvement efforts for several years now. "We use Six Sigma as our core methodology," reports Mary Cramer, master Six Sigma black belt and director for performance excellence at the five-campus health care system. "But our overriding philosophy is to bring whatever tool is appropriate to bear on a project." In fact, the teams at NYP regularly use lean management and other methodologies in addition to Six Sigma.

New York-Presbyterian's commitment to formal improvement methodologies for solving major problems has paid off in a big way by eliminating waste from the organization's emergency department processes. Members of performance improvement teams interviewed patients and clinicians in the organization's ED to understand how patient flow was working (and not working). Their study discovered that an average of 102 minutes elapsed from the time a patient entered the emergency room (if not brought in by an ambulance) until seen by a physician. The hospital's leaders agreed this waiting time was unacceptable. Staffers went to work on multiple fronts. They calculated the mean and median times for each step in ED visits for three types of patients—urgent, nonurgent, and fast track (i.e., patients presenting with minor conditions that did not require immediate attention from a clinical point of view).

The members of the process improvement team discovered a host of time-wasting bottlenecks in the ED patient visit process, including a long and cumbersome process for gathering information at patient registration. As a result, NYP implemented the use of computers on wheels (COWs) and changed work flow. Rather than going through all steps sequentially, processes were redesigned so that essential steps were tackled simultaneously whenever possible. As a result, the mean "door to doctor" time for an ED patient not arriving by ambulance has been cut from 102 minutes to under 50 minutes. Meanwhile, says Cramer, "Many pieces of information are being gathered at the bedside while patients are being seen by clinicians." Not surprisingly, patient satisfaction scores have improved considerably. The gains in efficiency have been sustained over time, and clinicians are also happier with the streamlined patient flow.

This same systematic approach to process improvement has been applied to other operations, including a largely neglected area with potential for high payoffs in efficiency and effectiveness—insertion of peripherally inserted central catheter (PICC) lines prior to patient discharge. Tony Dawson, NYP's vice president for quality and patient safety, explains. "Many of these lines are inserted in patients going home on long-term antibiotics, chemotherapy, or some sort of long-term infusion. A regular IV would not be comfortable. The PICC line can typically be used for months."

Most patients waiting for PICC line insertion are otherwise ready to be discharged. Members of the care team were aware that expensive delays occurred when discharge-ready patients were occupying beds while awaiting PICC line insertion. The problem was an amalgam of inefficiencies in patient flow, bed utilization, and patient satisfaction concern. Dawson and his colleagues were determined to solve this multifactor problem scientifically and analytically. They gathered data and found an average 2.4 day delay between order and insertion.

Further investigation uncovered a constellation of related issues. First, PICC line-insertion orders were often incomplete, requiring staff members to obtain additional information before they could move the process along. Second, the hospital had six different ways for ordering a PICC line insertion, which caused much confusion. Third, significant delays occurred for patients who required a diagnostic image for the PICC line insertion; radiology work flows were not formally integrated into the process. In short, Dawson notes, the entire PICC process was wasting a lot of resources and needed to be streamlined.

After the underlying process issues were uncovered, an interdisciplinary team created a single comprehensive method of physician ordering for PICC line insertion. The improved method mandated that all fields be filled so that incomplete orders could not be submitted. The order form was improved, and the accompanying informed consent form was also redesigned for precision and completeness. Additional ultrasound machines were purchased to speed patient flow through the diagnostic imaging process. As a result of these process improvements, bedside insertions increased from 47 percent before the initiative to 71 percent afterwards. The order-to-insertion time declined from 2.4 days to 1.3 days. Order compliance rose to 100 percent. The resulting improvements in resource utilization (i.e., reductions in waste) were substantial. Cramer says that successful reengineering of the PICC line-insertion process illustrates an important point about process improvement in hospital care. "While it's almost impossible for one project to tackle a global problem, like reducing overall lengths of stay, a hospital can make great gains by tackling dozens and dozens of smaller problems that underlie the big ones."

System-Wide Physician Performance Improvement: Fairview Health Services

Fairview Health Services (FHS), a seven hospital, integrated health system in Minneapolis-St. Paul, Minnesota, is one of several multihospital systems where leaders are formally integrating performance improvement into everyday business processes. With more than 300 employed physicians at 50 primary care sites and 37 specialty clinics, Fairview is participating in the CMS/Premier Hospital Quality Incentive Demonstration (HQID) project and is developing its own performance improvement programs as well. For example, in late 2004 and early 2005, FHS clinician executives devised a plan to improve physicians' quality performance. It used benchmark data from the Minnesota Community Measurement (MCM) program, a multistakeholder coalition (www.mnhealthcare.org).

Using MCM's physician quality-performance data, "We started with some good comparison data, and we weren't satisfied with our numbers at Fairview," recalls Barry Bershow, MD, FHS' medical director for quality and informatics. Beginning in 2005, Bershow and his colleagues developed quality performance improvement programs in several areas, including diabetes, hypertension, asthma, Chlamydia, obesity, and tobacco use. By 2007, the list of program areas had grown to 45.

The initiative's goal was to improve physician practices, individually and collectively, through a major internal pay for performance program. Essentially, Bershow says, "We went to the system's board of directors and said, 'What's it worth to you to have the best outcomes in the state?' They said it's worth a lot." So Bershow and his colleagues asked the board to allocate up to $15,000 per physician in the first year of the program, and the board agreed. The amount involved was quite significant. Had every single physician qualified for all potential payouts, the total would have been $4.5 million. Further, he notes, support from health plans added $350,000 to $400,000 in physician quality bonuses. Each physician had a potential for $17,270 in additional reimbursement—more than 10 percent of salary for primary care physicians.

The result? "The 10 percent salary boost for primary care physicians really did drive a lot of change," Bershow says. For example, at the beginning of 2005, only 3 percent of asthmatics had an asthma management program on file in their chart. By the end of the year, 80 percent did. Only 29 percent of sexually active, adult female patients were screened for Chlamydia in 2003–2004. Within the first year of Fairview's P4P program being implemented in 2005, that figure had jumped to 59 percent. It had reached 82 percent by late 2007. The program shows that payment can drive significant improvement and can do it in a relatively short time, according to Bershow. In fact, he says that the main problem with pay for performance programs has been a lack of significant funding. "When you hear the dollar amount that's being offered in most places" for physician performance improvement, he says, "it's just too paltry to drive change."

Another critical factor in the Fairview system's successes has been its robust, enterprise-wide electronic medical record (EMR) system. "I'm here to say pay for performance works very well, and it works best with an electronic medical record that can generate frequent, reliable reports," Bershow says. It is also crucial to base every guideline on the empirical clinical literature and to achieve strong physician buy-in through consensus building and data sharing. In the final analysis, Bershow concludes, the combination of gathering and presenting strong, clear data to physicians on a regular basis and linking outcomes measurement to pay has made a big difference at Fairview. "How do you separate the importance of frequent reports from the importance of the pay?" he asks. "Well, performance continues to improve in the areas where we have made payments, but it has stagnated or fallen backwards in areas where we haven't." The obvious conclusion, he says, is that clinicians respond to solid data and to reimbursement incentives, but performance improves the most when the two elements are combined in a robust, strategically focused program.

Cardiac Care Improvement: Hackensack Medical Center

One widely accepted clinical standard is 90 minutes to angioplasty, established by the American College of Cardiology (ACC). It requires moving an acute myocardial infarction (heart attack) patient from the ambulance and emergency room to the cardiac catheterization lab where an angioplasty balloon is inserted to restore normal blood flow, all in less than an hour and a half. A study suggests the 90-minute guideline is achieved less than half of the time (*Circulation*, 113(8):1079–1085). Hospital leaders are discovering that this clinical goal can only be accomplished with focused programs to maximize process efficiency.

Hackensack Medical Center in Hackensack, New Jersey, is one leading organization in which reworked processes have produced the desired results. The large teaching hospital has dramatically improved "door-to-balloon time" (and numerous other processes) within the hospital. Indeed, Hackensack's improvement work has been so successful that the hospital was the most highly rewarded participant in the CMS/Premier Hospital Quality Incentive Demonstration Project (HQID) last year. It received $744,000 in additional reimbursement from the Center for Medicare and Medicaid Services (CMS) for its achievements. This national recognition for excellence in performance improvement clearly demonstrates the multiple benefits for providers that are serious about efficiency and effectiveness.

Regina Berman, MA, administrator of performance improvement at Hackensack, provides background context for the organization's success. "We have spent a lot of time building reliable processes so that work becomes predictable and interwoven. Process standardization and integration have proven to be absolute preconditions for improving quality. To move from suboptimal performance to excellence, we used teams to examine the variations in process," Berman says. "They focused on modifying work flow to achieve what we called 'synchronicity of action.' The members of the teams reworked a series of interrelated processes to achieve a unified objective."

Charles Riccobono, MD, Hackensack's chief patient safety and quality officer, expands the point: "Where the current standard is to get the patient to the cath lab as quickly as possible and get circulation opened up to spare the muscle, it's all about getting the care team there in time. It really becomes a question of creating an efficient process." Several important, specific innovations were implemented with efficiency as the goal. First, those involved in the improvement effort isolated one major stumbling block: the way things had been done previously—someone would telephone the patient's primary care physician to ask which specialist should be called when the patient arrived in the emergency room. "We decided we couldn't waste time with that," says Riccobono. "So we developed a list of specialists who were already preferred by affiliated primary care physicians." Development of this preferential list, Berman adds, built trust between specialists and the hospital, and it improved efficiency by having all the updated contact information available for immediate use. Second, the hospital assigned a cardiologist to be on call for the emergency department, eliminating delays that had been a consistent problem prior to this performance improvement project.

The improvement team concurrently reworked the prehospital components of the total care package. Patients coming to the hospital by ambulance are now routinely given an electrocardiogram (EKG) while still in transit, which is read by an emergency physician in the ED. If the emergency physician confirms a heart attack diagnosis, the cath lab is called while the ambulance is still en route so that the cath lab staff can prepare for the patient's arrival. All these specific and coordinated changes have led to a significant door-to-balloon-time improvement.

According to Riccobono, the hospital now regularly achieves a 75-minute door-to-balloon time. Its overall composite score for performance is now 96.5 percent. The score encompasses several metrics, including time, administration of a beta blocker on arrival, and angioplasty treatment. By maximizing the efficiency of every aspect of this care process, the Hackensack team has also set a national standard for quality.

The evidence? "Our cardiac care number's terrific," says Riccobono. "You can't go anyplace in the country without bumping into our data."

VTE Prophylaxis:
Memorial Sloan-Kettering

An inpatient coming into the renowned Memorial Sloan-Kettering Cancer Center (MSKCC) in Manhattan would be expected to be at high risk for developing a deep-vein thrombosis, known technically as a venous thromboembolic event (VTE). The immobility of most cancer patients is a major cause of VTEs, and cancer itself can be a risk factor when it affects the patient's blood. Many patients coming to Memorial Sloan-Kettering are admitted for surgery, yet another risk factor. Other hospitals have created procedures for assessing VTE risk in incoming inpatients, but leaders at MSKCC decided a few years ago to assume all patients were at an elevated VTE risk and to act accordingly to minimize VTE occurrence.

MSKCC's clinician leaders created a two-pronged solution. They developed a rigorous protocol for VTE prophylaxis, and they reinforced it through the intelligent use of information technology. When a patient is admitted to MSKCC, the admitting physician uses the internally created, admissions-order template to create the appropriate orders for that patient's care. A VTE prophylaxis is a "forced order." The admitting physician is required to pick a drug and/or to order a mechanical compression device that will protect the patient against a VTE. The hospital's clinical leaders have chosen a low-molecular-weight heparin as the drug of choice for

VTE prophylaxis. The admitting physician can order the preferred drug (a specific generic chosen by physician consensus, with pharmacist guidance) or a subcutaneous heparin unless the patient has specific contraindications or exclusions.

This protocol was put in place in late 2006, after the order sets were built into the hospital's electronic medical record and clinical information system by a team of physicians led by David Artz, MD, medical director of information systems. However, says Jeremy Miransky, PhD, the organization's administrator for quality assessment and performance improvement, "We discovered some loopholes in the system. As a result, the organization's clinician leaders tightened the process. Now, if a physician does not order heparin for an incoming patient, the physician must explain why and document the reason. That move alone has created 100 percent compliance with the ordering sequence, and the vast majority of nonambulatory, presurgical patients receive prophylaxis."

A VTE prophylaxis optimization is just one example of many performance improvement and clinical-transformation projects at Memorial Sloan-Kettering. The organization's leaders are focused on opportunities to use evidence-based medicine practices to set the standards for quality and reduce operating costs. "The quality initiatives here stem from the belief that we should be working from objective, evidence-based medicine," Miransky says. For this reason, a protocol can only be added to the organization's performance criteria when it is shown to have the potential to improve patient care, to be easily measurable, to be readily explicable to individual physicians, and not to add significant human resources burdens.

The VTE prophylaxis-optimization program and others like it at MSKCC reflect another element in all the quality work there, namely, a strong use of information technology to support efficiency and effectiveness. "Automation is essential to achieve the economic improvements and clinical excellence we expect," says Dr. Artz. For example, Artz notes, MSKCC spends over $200 million a year in medications. "Standardization based on physician consensus in pharmaceutical practice reinforces selection of the less-costly medication that produces the desired therapeutic effect." The bottom line, though, remains care quality and patient safety. With the VTE prophylaxis protocol in place, MSKCC clinicians know they are averting potentially life-threatening medical errors and bringing a welcome standardization of top-quality medical practice across the organization.

Medical Group Performance Optimization: Hill Physicians Medical Group

California has long been the bellwether of change in medical care. The state is a vortex of health system turmoil, with constant shifts in reimbursement, finance, regulations, politics, and consumerism. One medical group has been a progressive leader in responding to the challenges: Hill Physicians Medical Group, a 2,800-doctor independent practice association (IPA) that serves over 350,000 patients from 1,600 office locations across nine big counties in the San Francisco Bay area and beyond. Founded in 1984, Hill Physicians has been a pioneer on many fronts in Northern California's intensely competitive, managed care-dominated marketplace. It has always approached the challenges with a spirit of creating the future, not preserving the past.

Those who know the organization weren't at all surprised when CEO Steve McDermott, a long-time leading
figure in California health care, became one of the prime
movers in the creation of the California pay for performance
program. It encompasses 35,000 physicians in 225 physician
organizations across the state, seven giant health plans, the
Pacific Business Group on Health, the Integrated Healthcare
Association, and a host of supporting organizations. That program paid more than $54 million in performance-based
bonuses to physicians in 2004.

McDermott and his colleagues have also developed a
far-reaching and sophisticated pay for performance program
for Hill Physicians. It distributes $35 million a year, a sum that
includes up to 20 percent of the annual pay of primary care
doctors. For specialists, the performance program typically
augments compensation between 5 percent and 10 percent of
compensation. "This is basically Business 101 applied to managing medical delivery systems," says McDermott. "It's not
rocket science. If you do it right and do it well, the doctors
respond positively."

Michael van Duren, MD, the group's vice president
of clinical services, adds, "We believe we should put our
money where our mouth is and actually pay for quality.
We've gotten to the point where 25 to 30 percent of compensation is at risk," generally believed to be the highest
at-risk compensation system for any medical group in the
country. "In fact," he says, "whenever we mention that figure, we get gasps. No one has ever said they could beat
that." For funding its pay for performance program, Hill
Physicians receive $5 million to $6 million each year from
health plans participating in the statewide program, but
the group pays a full $35 million a year in performance-
based income.

"To sustain this level of internal funding, we pay our primary care physicians 85 percent of RBRVS," van Duren says. (The Resource-Based Relative Value Scale is the foundation for physician reimbursement under Medicare.) "The 85 percent payout is a little bit less than the going rate for physicians services in the marketplace, but we say that it is fee for volume. Hill doctors can earn more than the going rate through performance as measured by the internal program. If you're about average in performance," he notes, "you get about 103 percent of RBRVS." The program measures doctors' efficiency ("for good stewardship of the managed care dollar," as van Duren puts it), a host of quality measures, and participation in educational programs. "We're very pleased with our program over the past five years," van Duren says. "People respect and trust it. Our quality scores go up year after year. And we're often listed as one of the top groups in northern California or the whole state."

What is the main lesson to be learned from this program? Rosaleen Derrington, Hill's chief medical services officer, says, "It actually has changed behavior. Four to five years ago, I can say that it was very difficult to get physicians to pay attention to these measures, especially the quality components. All the doctors thought they were already performing at very high levels of quality. But we've seen them buy in over time and steadily improve performance."

Everyone at Hill agrees that intelligent development and implementation of EMR systems will be needed to sustain the payment mechanism over the long run. Accordingly, the Hill Physicians Medical Group has been subsidizing half the cost of EMR implementation across its affiliated practice sites. Craig Lanway, the organization's vice president and CIO, reports that implementation has been slow, with only a few practices at a time going live with the three components of the EMR—the patient record itself, the practice management module, and document imaging (scanning). The first pilot sites went live with the EMR system in 2005. About 25 of the IPA's 1,600 practice sites had implemented the system by mid-2007. The process, Lanway concedes, will take years. Because it is an independent practice association (IPA), the organization cannot dictate terms to its member physicians. Every EMR installation must be successful in order to establish momentum toward the ultimate goal of system-wide implementation.

Hill's executives and clinician leaders hope their EMR rollout will also facilitate growth of an innovative case-management program for high-risk populations. This proactive program, van Duren says, will receive a strong boost once more practices are using the organization's full EMR. Certainly, capitated payment in the local market has been a spur to develop such innovative programs at Hill Physicians. But the nature of payment can also be constraining. "In a way," McDermott says, "managed care has connected us more with the health plans. Many American providers are focused on 'doing what's right for the patient,' but they are not conscious of the broader impact. Here, we don't lose sight of what's right for individual patients, but we're much more conscious of the broader community and population contexts as well."

Tying It All Together

The imperatives to become efficient and effective certainly reflect the broader context. These case studies identify many different reasons for reducing costs and producing top quality. They also show that individual performance improvement programs can produce impressive gains in both efficiency and effectiveness. Providers do not need one program for cutting costs and another for improving quality. Indeed, strategic commitments to improving performance across the enterprise can jump-start a plethora of benefits in hospitals, medical groups, and health systems. The next chapter takes an executive-level look at the performance improvement methodologies that produce the desired outcomes.

| SIX |

PERFORMANCE IMPROVEMENT METHODOLOGIES TO ORGANIZE AND MANAGE CHANGE

Hospitals and medical groups that have made huge strides forward in optimizing efficiency and effectiveness have used formal methodologies for achieving desired results. In contrast to organizations that have not yet managed to minimize the costs of producing consistently top-quality medical services, trail-blazing organizations in the medical marketplace have embraced strategically proven techniques for performance improvement (PI). Health care's leaders in efficiency and effectiveness are fortunate to be able to get right to work—once their organization decides to respond to the imperatives—with a variety of PI tools that have already led to remarkable progress in other industries and work well "out of the box" in health care.

This chapter discusses general principles for choosing PI tools that mesh with an organization's culture, and it presents a list of the general methodologies that have worked well for progressive hospitals and medical groups. Although some organizations might be able to solve cost and quality problems without selecting a management technique or two to guide the process, an unstructured approach is not recommended. The organizationally appropriate PI tool(s) to institutionalize efficiency and effectiveness should be chosen in consideration of historical experiences, both positive and negative.

Positive Benefits

Even a cursory glance at the case studies in the preceding chapter provides several reasons for selecting a proven methodology for managing the necessary changes in organizational performance.

- Tools with a track record (i.e., those supported by how-to books that have sold well and an array of articles linking them to successes in a variety of industries) provide a common understanding of the process that will be followed across the enterprise. They are, in effect, the same page from which everyone should be singing.

- Because proven PI tools have been tested and refined in many organizational environments, they are already tailored to the demands of making systemic changes in dynamic marketplaces. They will provide much-needed confidence in the process because stakeholders will know they have already worked well in comparable settings.

- The tools give sound initial guidance for defining appropriate investments in staffing, training, education, and information technology. Because the leading PI tools have evolved over many years—none of them being really new—they help prevent under-investment in managerial and clinical areas that are critical to success.

- Because they are data-rich and data-driven, these tools generally provide useful performance benchmarks for getting started. Organizations that use objective data as required by the processes are much more likely to make appropriate adjustments that will lead to success. They will become "learning organizations" if they have not already achieved this important organizational characteristic.

Negative Knowledge

In the important sense of negative knowledge—knowing what *not* to do—the proven PI tools have developed over the years to prevent problems that have plagued narrowly focused "quality improvement" projects in health care organizations for many years. Most of the programs in vogue in the 1980s and 1990s failed because they did not incorporate the comprehensive mechanisms that are built into today's performance improvement and clinical transformation tools.

- They did not enforce unswerving commitment and direct involvement from the top of the organization. The failures of PI "lite" projects can often be attributed to lack of time and money invested by the board, CEO, medical staff leaders, and executive management-level support.

- The unsuccessful programs tended to focus narrowly on specific "mechanical" problems, such as streamlining the admitting process or reducing waiting times for diagnostic tests. They did not recognize or address the fundamental interconnectedness of all the processes involved in the care of each patient.

- They were not explicitly linked to an organization's vision, mission, or strategic business goals. Consequently, they almost never became core values that permeated the enterprise and defined the corporate culture across all disciplines. They did not establish "this is how we do things here" in any special way that defined the organization.

- The narrow, single-function improvement programs almost always fell short in providing needed data and IT support. Consequently, they did not generate the extensive information needed to coordinate ongoing changes for accomplishing quantified goals.

- The unsuccessful programs often resulted in little more than disappointments and, even worse, layoffs. Employees became quickly disenchanted with single-function PI programs because they tended to do more harm than good in the final analysis. These programs became true examples of the uninspiring adage, "The more things change, the more they stay the same."

In summary, most of the previous performance improvement efforts in patient care organizations were not properly embedded in a comprehensive organizational context. They tended to lack the broad conceptual foundations of the performance methodologies that have matured in other industries over the past 50 years. And without the information systems now available in health care, many of these initiatives ground to a data-starved halt long before anything of lasting value was accomplished.

Lessons from the Case Studies

Although the case studies in the previous chapter clearly show how PI tools and IT infrastructure can reduce the costs of producing top-quality health care, they also lead to some helpful observations about the improvement process. For example, Christina Saint Martin, vice president for governance and administration at Virginia Mason Medical Center in Seattle, describes the organization's six-year journey to select and implement the Toyota Production System (TPS). Once the leaders became convinced that its concepts could be successfully grafted into all aspects of day-to-day operations of a major hospital and its medical staff, they made a complete commitment to TPS. Most importantly, Saint Martin says, "VMMC's full embrace of TPS went far beyond the use of a toolkit." Virginia Mason initially and unapologetically chose TPS to save the organization after a few financially disastrous years in the late 1990s.

But in the process of using TPS to respond to market trends and to improve its bottom line, Saint Martin and her colleagues discovered that the methodology had produced many other improvements, from reworking nurse staffing to reducing central-line infections and ventilator-acquired pneumonia. They found the entire way of doing things at Virginia Mason was transformed by the Toyota methodology. "The TPS paradigm is really changing the culture," Saint Martin says. "Having looked at change throughout our health system's history, particularly at what has worked and what hasn't, we realized that change was going to have to be drastic to achieve meaningful results. So, going 'whole hog' was absolutely necessary. Piecemeal change wasn't going to achieve what we wanted to achieve." Hospitals all across the country should be prepared to make a similar, serious commitment in order to accomplish an equally impressive transformation. Virginia Mason is a world-class role model.

Enterprise-wide change has also been at the core of performance improvement efforts launched in the past several years at New York-Presbyterian Hospital, reports Mary Reich Cooper, MD, JD, the organization's vice president and chief quality officer. When the 1998 merger of New York Hospital and Presbyterian Hospital created the largest not-for-profit, nonsectarian hospital in the United States, the organization had been using a self-developed "Plan-Do-Check-Act (PDCA) model called PRIDE," she reports, but it was replaced enterprise-wide with Six Sigma, "to drive change throughout the organization." In the last couple of years, the organization has also begun using lean management principles for some purposes, especially for broad process-change efforts.

Dr. Cooper believes that any of the widely used PI methodologies will produce desired outcomes if used correctly and applied vigorously, as old and incomplete processes are replaced with new processes that are evidence-based, data driven, and collaborative. In fact, Cooper says, it is no coincidence that a huge academic medical center like hers has chosen to accomplish desired changes with data-driven performance improvement methodologies like Six Sigma and lean. The key lies in achieving the buy-in of physicians, who are data-focused scientists. "Not only do the physicians have to lead the process. They need to see that it is based in sound science," she notes. "There's a science of safety that's been demonstrated with nuclear reactors, oil tankers, and all sorts of high-risk industries. We used this knowledge with our Six

Sigma rollout, focusing on a scientific approach to change with appropriate data use," she says. "We've consistently tried to frame our PI within a scientific perspective, and it's gone well. We teach it in the same way we try to teach the diagnosis of pneumonia."

Careful attention to scientific principles is clearly one of the reasons that New York-Presbyterian has been so successful in maintaining the medical staff's commitment to efficiency and effectiveness throughout the organization. It is an essential consideration for successful selection and use of any PI tool. Progressive provider organizations have been able to achieve successful, physician-supported transformation with several different models. The next section reviews these proven PI methodologies for leaders who need to know what needs to be done, but not how to do it, to become efficient and effective throughout their organizations.

Lean Management

In their pioneering book, *Lean Thinking* (Simon & Schuster, 2003), James P. Womack and Daniel T. Jones defined a set of five basic principles that characterize a lean enterprise. According to Womack and Jones, lean organizations:

1. Specify value from the standpoint of the end customer by product family.
2. Identify all the steps in the value stream for each product family, eliminating every step and every action and every practice that does not create value.
3. Make the remaining value-creating steps occur in a tight and integrated sequence so the product will flow smoothly toward the customer.
4. As flow is introduced, let customers pull value from the next upstream activity.

5. As these steps lead to greater transparency, enabling managers and teams to eliminate further waste, pursue perfection through continuous improvement.

Lean's key elements are eliminating waste in production processes and redirecting human effort toward value-added activities. Lean principles go back to Kiichiro Toyoda's founding of the Toyota Production System in the auto industry.

> As Kiichiro Toyoda, Taiichi Ohno, and others at Toyota looked at...[auto production problems] in the 1930s, and more intensely just after World War II, it occurred to them that a series of simple innovations might make it more possible to provide both continuity in process flow and a wide variety in product offerings. They therefore revisited [Henry] Ford's original thinking and invented the Toyota Production System. This system in essence shifted the focus of the manufacturing engineer from individual machines and their utilization to the flow of the product through the total process.[1]

Significantly, the concept of flow became the foundation of optimized production and the basis for lean management principles. Lean also recognizes how management engineering can transform traditional production methods that have allowed waste to accumulate over time. In health care, provider organizations have used lean principles to approach and attack many systemic problems. For example, the case studies in Chapter 5 include several examples of lean applications that optimized clinician work flow by analyzing every

---

1. These comments are from a concise history presented at www.lean.org/WhatsLean/History.cfm on the Lean Enterprise Institute's website.

step in a complex process (e.g., medication management), reengineering the processes to eliminate waste and add value, and eliminating all systemic causes of medical errors.

A variety of organizations have arisen recently to spread lean principles in health care. One of them, Ireland-based Lean Healthcare Services, presents a concise summary of the essence of lean thinking as applied to health care (www.lean-healthcareservices.com/leanexplained02.htm):

- Eliminate waste through understanding the value to the patient and how to deliver that value

- Create an efficient and waste-free continuous flow system built on a pull vs. 'batch and queue' approach

- Continually pursue a perfect system

The organization's website also includes a useful list of examples of waste common to production processes in health care:

- Redundant capture of information on admission

- Multiple recording of patient information

- Excess supplies stored in multiple locations

- Time spent looking for charts

- Patient waiting rooms

- Continuous back-tracking of movement of medical staff

- Time spent waiting for equipment, lab results, x-rays, etc.

- Time spent dealing with complaints about service

These are the types of waste that are eliminated with lean management. Readers who want to develop a deeper knowledge of lean management and its applications will find ample resources simply by doing a web search on the key words *lean management*. (The *Wikipedia* coverage presents a useful summary.) Most of the examples will come from industries other than health care. However, the principles are universal, and health care can learn a lot by studying how waste has been eliminated in other high-tech, high-touch industries.

Toyota Production System

Although lean management principles are applied in most major industries and have begun to prove their worth in patient-care organizations, they have their clear origins in the Toyota Production System created for the manufacture of Toyota automobiles. Lean management principles are commonly studied and taught separately from the Toyota Production System (TPS), but the two schools remain closely linked in theory and in practice. Thus, books, articles, speakers, and seminars often deal with both. For example, *Becoming Lean: Inside Stories of U.S. Manufacturers* (Productivity Press, 1998), edited by Jeffrey K. Liker, PhD, deals with both.

In Chapter 2 of this book, "Bringing the Toyota Production System to the United States: A Personal Perspective," John Y. Shook outlines core principles of TPS:

- *Jidoka*: a Japanese word meaning "building-in quality and designing operations and equipment so that people are not tied to machines but are free to perform value-added work that is appropriate for humans"
- *Just-in-time*: "the right part at the right time in the right amount"
- *One-piece flow* for maximum efficiency
- *Takt time*: a concept that helps create just-in-time production

Translating these concepts into medical services requires careful thought and focused work. However, general concepts such as streamlining work flow processes and creating value through individual work contributions are being applied in a variety of health care settings. At Virginia Mason Medical Center, a great deal of work has been successfully focused on eliminating waste in the production of patient-care services and eliminating medical errors through the TPS. The Toyota Production System is obviously a valuable tool in the hands of dedicated health care providers. From our perspective, the issue is not choosing between lean and TPS, but simply choosing one and getting to work with it.

Six Sigma

Six Sigma is another set of principles and practices that is moving successfully into the health care industry after proving its value in other major industries. The online encyclopedia, *Wikipedia*, provides a good introduction:

> Six Sigma is a set of practices originally developed by Motorola to systematically improve processes by eliminating defects...While the particulars of the methodology were originally formulated by Bill Smith at Motorola in 1986, Six Sigma was heavily inspired by six preceding decades of quality improvement methodologies such as quality control, TQM [Total Quality Management], and Zero Defects. Like its predecessors, Six Sigma asserts the following:
> - A continuous effort to reduce variation in process outputs is key to business success.
> - Manufacturing and business processes can be measured, analyzed, improved, and controlled.

- Succeeding at achieving sustained quality improvement requires commitment from the entire organization, particularly from top-level management.

Wikipedia also notes that "Six Sigma," a registered service mark and trademark of Motorola, Inc., is a statistical term referring to processes that operate at defect levels below 3.4 defects per one million opportunities.

In health care, Six Sigma is being used to solve a variety of problems involving wasted resources (including time) and substandard quality. In an informative online article entitled "Measuring Six Sigma Results in the Healthcare Industry" (http://healthcare.isixsigma.com/library/content/c040623a.asp), Carolyn Pexton notes:

The following represent some of the successful projects and initiatives taking place at hospitals and health systems throughout the United States, applying a combination of Six Sigma, lean, and change management methods:

- Projects at Thibodaux Regional Medical Center in Louisiana have yielded more than $4 million in revenue growth, cash flow improvement, and cost savings.
- Good Samaritan Hospital in Los Angeles reduced registry expenses by mapping multiple process drivers and achieved cost savings between $5.5 and $6 million.
- Virtua Health in New Jersey has had a vigorous Six Sigma program in place for several years as part of their Star Initiative to achieve operational excellence. In one project focused on congestive heart failure, length of stay was reduced from six to four days; patient education improved from 27 to 80

percent; and chart consistency improved from 67 to 93 percent.

- Valley Baptist Health System in Harlingen, Texas, reduced surgical cycle time, adding capacity for an additional 1,100 cases per year and increasing potential revenue more than $1.3 million annually.
- Boston Medical Center improved throughput in diagnostic imaging, with a potential impact of more than $2.2 million in cost savings and revenue growth.
- The Women and Infants Hospital of Rhode Island successfully used Six Sigma and change management to standardize operating procedures for embryo transfer, yielding a 35 percent increase in implantation rates.

According to Pexton, health care organizations are mixing and combining a variety of approaches to process improvement in order to achieve the best results. Few are only using Six Sigma, lean management, or the Toyota Production System. Although we generally favor using a single methodology for becoming efficient and effective, a combination of two or more PI tools is fine—if one tool does not quite provide the impetus that an organization needs to move forward and if the integration of more than one tool does not delay getting started.

Plan-Do-Check-Act/Balanced Scorecard

Our research also found health care organizations that are successfully using an established variation on Six Sigma, "Plan-Do-Check-Act" (PDCA). Again, *Wikipedia* provides a helpful, well-synthesized summary of the concept (at http://en.wikipedia. org/wiki/PDCA).

PDCA was made popular by Dr. W. Edwards Deming, who is considered by many to be the father of modern quality control; however it was always referred to by him as the 'Shewhart cycle.' Later in Deming's career, he modified PDCA to 'Plan, Do, Study, Act' (PDSA) so as to better describe his recommendations. In Six Sigma programs, this cycle is called 'Define, Measure, Analyze, Improve, Control' (DMAIC). . . . PDCA should be repeatedly implemented, as quickly as possible, in upward spirals that converge on the ultimate goal, each cycle closer than the previous. This approach is based on the understanding that our knowledge and skills are always limited, but improving as we go. Often, key information is unknown, or unknowable. Rather than enter 'analysis paralysis' to get it perfect the first time, it is better to be approximately right than exactly wrong. Over time and with better knowledge and skills, PDCA will help define the ideal goal, as well as help get us there.

In health care, PDCA principles have been used in numerous instances in the context of the Balanced Scorecard (BSC) approach, which analyzes mission and strategy into objectives organized according to financial, customer, internal business process, and learning and growth perspectives. In *Managed Care Magazine* (www.managedcaremag.com/archives/0309/ 0309.peer_balanced.pdf), Judith A. Shutt described the use of PDCA within a Balanced Scorecard initiative pursued by Duke Children's Hospital (DCH):

In 1997, the average length of stay at DCH was eight days, or 20 percent longer than the national average. The average per-patient cost at DCH was $15,000 (more money than was being reimbursed); consequently, the hospital was faced with a projected $7 million increase in annual losses within four years. It was apparent that drastic measures had to be initiated quickly to preserve financial stability. The BSC was identified as the one management strategy that linked the four areas—finance, customer satisfaction, business processes, and staff satisfaction—and appeared to be the answer regarding both short- and long-term improvements.

After defining the organization's management requirements for meeting goals, the medical director began the implementation of the BSC in the pediatric intensive care unit (PICU). Within six months, the PICU reduced the cost per case by 12 percent and increased patient satisfaction by 8 percent. Reorganization, new protocols, and an emphasis on 'multidisciplinary teams focused on a particular illness or disease' were credited for the improvements. By 2000, the BSC was evidence throughout DCH, and the hospital successfully lowered its cost per case by $5,000, leading to a net gain of $4 million.

Although the organizations featured in Chapter 5 did not use PDCA and BSC as often as other techniques, both were clearly productive tools when used separately or in combination. A provider organization should not be dissuaded from using them if its managers or consultants have the skills to achieve desired results with PDCA and/or BSC. Moving forward right away with a PI tool that works is far more important than waiting for the perfect tool.

Expert Consensus: Tools for Changing the Future

Experts in the various PI methodologies have their biases, but they tend to agree on one important point. For business organizations in any industry to apply PI methodologies successfully, the enterprise needs to do so strategically. Leaders must be committed to making changes and reallocating resources for the explicit purpose of creating a desired future, different from the future likely to occur if nothing changed. The requisite changes include creating new cultures and new ways of thinking. The proven PI tools are meant to create big transformations across the enterprise, not to "fix" small, discrete problems within a broader context of business as usual.

Experts also tend to agree on the importance of flexibility. As Jeffrey Liker says about *The Toyota Way: 14 Management Principles from the World's Greatest Manufacturer* (McGraw-Hill, 2004), "One of the things I was trying to accomplish with *The Toyota Way* was to counterbalance the concept of the idea of Lean as a toolkit. I think that whole way of thinking that there is something you can just pick up as a set of tools to 'Lean out' a system, is a misunderstanding of the Toyota process. The reality is that lean was an abstraction from observing Toyota, and that abstraction has been converted into a lot of different variations and flavors, which are being deployed en masse to many, many different kinds of businesses, and these things are very variable."

Asked how organizations outside auto manufacturing (including health care) can successfully apply lean management principles, Liker says that "The most important thing is that leadership from the top be both consistent and patient over the long term. If the leaders are consistent and patient, they will have success. And whether they use Kaizen workshops, value-stream mapping, or pilot projects, they will find success over time, if the leadership is right." Certainly, Liker notes, the unusual incentive misalignments in health care—particularly the fact that most physicians work in hospitals but not for hospitals—pose special problems in health care. But the key to progress is long-term leadership and a holistic approach to change.

Success is only possible with a long-term, enterprise-wide embrace of process change that becomes fully embedded in the corporate culture. Gary Convis, recently retired president of Toyota Motor Manufacturing Kentucky, Inc., agrees. "My honest opinion is that culture is so much more important than people realize," Convis says. "Most people don't even put it on the road map or recognize it as a critical component of how to get better. But I was with Toyota 24 years, and in my first two weeks in Japan in 1984, I could sense that I was encountering a culture that was not like anything I'd ever experienced before. The reality is that if you're going to make any kind of change to an organization, culture is a foundational issue."

The good news for health care executives, Convis says, is that TPS concepts are flexible and "totally, totally translatable" to medical care provider organizations. "TPS," he says, "is about thinking and philosophy, and there are many, many ways to apply those philosophies to different subjects." In fact, Convis says, the complex details of patient-care processes share similarities with some auto manufacturing processes. He has compared the processes of arc welding and preventing ventilator-acquired pneumonia. To be done correctly, both require professional attention to details like coordinating resources, positioning materials, and controlling their use with predictable precision. In the end, Convis says, "It usually comes back to consistency of leadership and priorities. We've been blessed with a leadership at Toyota that has always had a certain philosophy and lived it." The same lesson can surely be applied to efficiency and effectiveness in health care.

PI Is About Learning and Empowerment

Finally, the proven PI tools recognize the need for employees to work together in highly complex environments. Complexity is unquestionably the norm in health care. The science and technology of medical care are always changing, and currently changing faster than ever before. The executives and health professionals who use PI tools need to learn to adapt them to constantly changing circumstances. They need to know the "rules of the game" and how to perform as a team.

All of the effective PI tools require ongoing, enterprise-wide education that teaches everyone how to recognize and solve problems collaboratively. Consequently, because workers are well trained, they are empowered to call a halt when they see a problem that could lead to a production error. They are also empowered to make changes that will prevent the problem from occurring again, in contrast to health care's longstanding practice of finding "work-arounds" instead. Executives who are leading the implementation of PI in their organizations should make sure that they select a methodology that educates and empowers personnel to do the right things, all the time. When this philosophy becomes part of the corporate culture, the enterprise is positioned to meet the imperatives for efficiency and effectiveness in all that it does.

Additional Observations from a Site Visit

Anyone lucky enough to take a tour of Toyota Corporation's plant in Georgetown, Kentucky, will not regret the time spent. For an hour, a friendly tour guide speaks through an electronic device into visitors' headsets, as an electric tram wheels visitors through dozens of work areas. The 18-year-old, 7.5-million-square-foot plant (the largest Toyota facility in the world) employs 7,000 workers and produces 500,000 Toyota cars every year. It is a 21st-century beehive of activity and a fascinating place to explore.

The Georgetown plant is exceptionally efficient in use of human resources, and its overall automation is highly impressive. But what strikes a visitor most is the conscious quality of operations and management here; the thoughtfulness and purposefulness of it. Quality principles have been built into every work process, and every Toyota employee has been indoctrinated in a culture of quality. The combination of a fierce commitment to quality, a zero-defects philosophy, and a conscious approach to every process, has helped propel Toyota to global leadership in auto sales and a worldwide reputation across industries.

The Toyota Production System has several characteristics that are instructive for health care providers:

- Corporate leaders have created a sustainable philosophy around their mission and have set goals for operations accordingly.

- The core philosophy is founded on a culture of quality, excellence, striving for improvement, teamwork, and inquiry.

- Everything is examined and questioned, and a body of employees, given a democratic voice in promoting change, continuously improves objective processes.

- Leaders nurture a learning organization—one that continually transforms to meet customer needs and expectations.

Of course, many comprehensive books are available on Toyota's recipe for success, including *The Toyota Way* by Jeffrey K. Liker (McGraw-Hill, 2004) and *Creating Lean Corporations: Reengineering from the Bottom Up to Eliminate Waste,* by Jeffrey Morgan (Productivity Press, 2005). The specific details of the Toyota Production System and of lean management are far beyond the scope of this chapter.

So, why can't health care delivery work like this? Had one posed this question to hospital executives 10 years ago, the "obvious" responses would have been: 1) delivering care to patients in hospitals is nothing like producing consumer goods like cars; and 2) health care could never, in any way, resemble any industry like the automotive industry. Fortunately, a growing number of progressive executives and clinical leaders across the United States has decided in the past decade that health care can be produced along similar lines. In fact, these leaders have been aggressively studying performance improvement techniques and applying them to health care delivery.

An Altered Landscape

The work of today's pioneering health care organizations is not evolving in a vacuum. The industry's progressive organizations, including those featured in Chapter 5, are pushing health care to become more like other industries—in other words, to become more customer responsive. At the same time, purchasers, payers, and consumers are demanding greater value, and the mainstream news media feature dramatic stories on gaps in the quality of care. Wrong-side surgeries, medication error-caused deaths, and other reports of bad care resonate with a public fearful of substandard care.

Such fears are not irrational. Numerous reports have highlighted embarrassing statistics about wasteful and dangerous deficiencies in the delivery of health care. Outsiders are raising public awareness of quality problems and forcing providers to respond in public. Fortunately, many providers have responded with industry-wide initiatives that promote improvement in individual organizations. For example, the CMS/Premier Hospital Quality Incentive Demonstration (HQID) project, the largest and most visible pay for performance initiative in the hospital industry, has been demonstrating exceptional results since its inception a few years ago. In January 2007, leaders of the program announced that the 260 participating hospitals raised overall quality by 11.8 measured percentage points in two years, based on their delivery of 30 nationally standardized and widely accepted care measures to patients in five clinical areas. Quality variation between top and bottom performers continued to shrink, and every hospital in the program documented measurable quality improvement.

Richard A. Norling, Premier's president and CEO, reflects on the program's success. "I think it has happened because participating hospitals have used the demonstration to accelerate or jump-start quality improvement," he says. "I also think that most of the hospitals felt this was the logical extension of a very significant trend started by the Center for Medicare and Medicaid Services (CMS). Key to the success," he adds, "are a healthy dose of 'I'll-show-you'-type competition among the hospitals and a new spirit of collaboration between all the stakeholders."

Donald M. Berwick, MD, president and CEO at the Institute for Healthcare Improvement (IHI), underscored a

positive implication of the overall results when he comment-
ed on the progress made to date in a January 2007 statement
following the release of findings after two years of development: "The main point is that the majority of hospitals in the
HQID project, even those on the lower end of the scale,
improved their quality of care across the board with respect
to reliable use of scientifically based practices. Hospitals want
to offer high quality care," Berwick added. "Sometimes they
just need to be pointed in the right direction. The HQID
project has offered hospitals a guideline to improve their
patient care."

Given the successes of several initiatives and the
increasing availability of data to the public, providers are less
able to hide behind the old excuses of customer ignorance
and lack of data and information. The rising costs of health
care and the increasing shift of payment responsibility to
patients are also making the status quo unsustainable. The old
reasons for not acting are now weak and disappearing.
Perhaps, most importantly, the growing number of successes
in cost reduction and quality improvement put real pressure
on the many hospitals that have not yet responded to the
imperatives.

The Power of Opportunity

Some providers have embraced performance improvement,
not because they were financially imperiled, but because they
saw opportunity in being better. Bronson Methodist Hospital
in Kalamazoo, Michigan, and North Mississippi Medical
Center (NMMC) in Tupelo provide excellent examples of
this trend because both have received the Malcolm Baldrige
National Quality Award—Bronson in 2005 and NMMC in
2006. Winners in this competition are not just the tops in

their own industries. Recipients of the Baldrige Award enter the ranks of the most efficient and effective companies in the United States.

According to Michele Serbenski, Bronson Healthcare Group's executive director of corporate effectiveness and customer satisfaction, meeting the Baldrige criteria was key, not only to winning the award, but to all the innovations she and her colleagues have been able to implement at Bronson. (Ms. Serbenski's title itself is an indicator of her organization's progressive orientation.) "The Baldrige criteria force you to formalize and define your approach to everything," she says. "I think that Bronson is a successful organization because we truly aspire to be excellent. And so we have aligned everything that we do around that goal, from our vision to be a national leader in health care quality to our three corporate strategies—clinical excellence, corporate effectiveness, and customer and service excellence." The organization works off a simple, clear, one-page Plan for Excellence that makes the commitment clear to everyone. "We really have a 'raise the bar' culture that begins with our CEO. You achieve something, and you continually strive to be better. Once you achieve something, you say, great, now, how do we get better?"

Charles Stokes, CEO at North Mississippi, describes the quest for quality in the context of a constellation of strategic organizational goals. "Our focus has been on five critical success factors: people, service, quality, financial, and growth," he says. All lead to intensive work in continuous quality improvement, financial strength, and revenue growth. "I think we were a recipient [of the Baldrige Award]," he says, "because of our ability to focus on those five critical success factors and produce measurable results in every area. Baldrige provides a framework for us to focus on things that are important." It also emphasizes data and objectivity. Stokes credits a data-focused emphasis as one of the most significant elements in his hospital's success.

North Mississippi has used PDCA (Plan–Do–Check–Act) and Six Sigma as core methodologies for bringing about quality improvement and other changes. Other hospitals have achieved comparable success with Toyota, lean, and other improvement processes discussed in this chapter. The take-home point is not to find which one is the best, but to find the one that works in each individual organization. The importance of making a choice is obvious in the following review of factors that are common to the success of organizations that have used different tools to become models of efficiency and effectiveness.

| SEVEN |

ORGANIZATIONAL SUCCESS FACTORS FOR EFFICIENCY AND EFFECTIVENESS

The case studies in Chapter 5 and the overview of process improvement techniques in Chapter 6 contain valuable information about organizational characteristics of provider organizations that have become efficient and effective in their daily operations. Drawing on information from the case study interviews, this chapter lists the success factors of hospitals and medical groups that are leading the industry in responses to the marketplace's new imperatives. The list is also based on the authors' many years of consulting (Bauer) and journalistic (Hagland) interactions with organizations pursuing performance improvement and clinical transformation.

Leaders can use this chapter as a checklist to make plans and gauge progress for their own enterprises. It identifies attributes of organizations that have succeeded in setting top-level standards for quality, reducing the costs of operations, and reallocating resources to meet strategic goals. This chapter is short and to the point with the intent of helping leaders focus their actions by highlighting the critical success factors (CSF). Leaders should already know how to take action and/or have staff that can get the job done, once the CSFs are identified and fully integrated into organizational culture.

Below are seven proven criteria to guide the overall process of responding to the new imperatives. Hospitals and medical groups may need to expand the list to encompass special dimensions of their particular mission and vision. However, all items listed in this chapter need to remain on the checklist. The case studies were selected to represent the gamut of providers—for-profit and tax-exempt, large and small, urban and rural, etc.—and the leaders were doing all these things.

Standardization

Successful organizations have been willing and able to develop standards for guiding and measuring production processes. Their leaders constantly seek to eliminate one of the major causes of poor quality and unnecessary cost in any industry — variability in production. A rich management literature shows how serious problems are created when employees dedicated to the same task are allowed to use different methods, tools, and/or supplies. The same literature also shows how management engineering determines the least-cost combination of resources that produces a product of defined quality—the bottom of the U-shaped cost curves from economic analysis.

Production managers are taught how to push toward the bottom of the cost curve because any other combination of inputs or processes is, by definition, wasteful. Getting there requires managers to set and enforce measurable standards for doing a job the right way with the right tools. Standards are not just for manufacturing, either. They are equally important in service industries where lives are on the line, as demonstrated by the phenomenal improvements made in commercial aviation when airline manufacturers started putting uniform instrumentation in cockpits, and airlines started teaching all pilots to fly planes the same way.

The same principles were applied to the administration of anesthetics, making modern anesthesia as safe as flying. The case studies in this book showed impressive gains obtained by applying the same principles to many other clinical services. The case for promoting standardization in health care is unambiguous. Of course, resistance to standardization is equally certain because physicians and nurses have been trained in so many different ways and have become accustomed to so many different products. Leaders must resist pleas to maintain the old way of doing things when the new standard is implemented. Multiple standards are inefficient. A standard should be flexible (see the next section), but it should be *the* standard.

The case studies clearly demonstrate the need to put appropriate clinicians in charge of standardization, giving them authority, accountability, and resources to eliminate the waste that flows from unnecessary variation in production. Standardization will not necessarily be easy, but it is absolutely essential for providers who plan to finance growth through savings. Board members, ultimately accountable for the wise management of organizational resources, should put top priority on working with senior executives and clinical leaders to make standardization part of the corporate culture.

Flexibility

Efficiency and effectiveness are moving targets in health care. The optimal way to produce any given medical service evolves constantly with the development of new drugs and devices, the publication of new research results, and changes in the payment system. Consequently, standards need to be flexible. A standard that defines today's best combination of inputs for producing a service of predetermined quality is unlikely to be the constant standard for years to come. Some standards will require only minor modification over time, while others will need to be dramatically restructured.

Groups responsible for standards need to be given permanent status and ongoing authority to change with the times. (Of course, organizational change should be strategic, that is, initiated in anticipation of environmental changes, as described in Chapter 1.) Performance improvement and clinical transformation programs cannot be organized as "one-shot" activities to be disbanded as soon as standards are promulgated. In all but the smallest organizations, departments or divisions created to pursue efficiency and effectiveness will need to become part of the permanent organizational structure. Consultants will be appropriate substitutes for internal resources in many situations, especially for initiating PI activities. If maintaining an internal PI resource does not make sense, then cost-effective, long-term contracts for services from qualified consultants should be pursued.

Whatever the best solution for a particular organization, the CSF here is providing resources to support continual revision of standards in accord with changes in medical science and technology. Active involvement in progressive professional associations and periodic participation in standards-focused meetings will also be important. Few, if any, provider organizations can reach the economies of scale to be self-sufficient in meeting the changing criteria for efficiency and effectiveness. Fortunately, as demonstrated in the case studies in Chapter 5, most organizations that have the resources for do-it-yourself specification of standards are active in national organizations and conferences. Leaders from organizations with more limited resources can benefit immensely by interacting with their counterparts from benchmark institutions by belonging to the national organizations and attending relevant meetings. It's a cost-effective way to stay flexible and respond to the imperatives.

Integration

The national leaders in cost and quality have highly integrated organizations, beginning with information technology. Networked hardware and software are the norm because efficiency and effectiveness can only be built on a foundation of shared data and common IT platforms. Broadband connectivity facilitates practitioners' access to patient data from all locations and timely interaction with all support systems. Systems are interactive. Information flows seamlessly between the clinic, operations, and finance. State-of-the-art network security regulates access, protects integrity, and assures availability of the data when and where they are needed.

The national leaders in efficiency and effectiveness tend to be multi-institution organizations. Several providers have come together as a business enterprise to create economies of scale in infrastructure, such as integrated IT systems. Although most of these organizations are single corporate entities created by mergers and acquisitions, formal affiliation agreements can also create business partnerships that achieve economies of scale. Outsourcing arrangements and provider–vendor partnerships have proven to be viable alternatives to mergers.

Two qualifications are important to the discussion of integration. First, mergers to create multi-institutional systems can go too far, creating diseconomies of scale. Astute leaders recognize the need to create systems that are big enough to afford necessary infrastructure—but not so big that they are unmanageable. Second, outsourcing does not necessarily mean that work will be done in another country. Significant economic advantages can often be gained by exporting some activities to "offshore" workers and computers located in other countries, but domestic outsourcing can also produce significant economic benefits. The CSF is integration. Providers can work out the details of integration in several different ways.

Alignment

Alignment might seem like another word for integration, but the two concepts are different. Some highly integrated delivery systems are inefficient and ineffective because the stakeholders are not aligned. Alignment requires that everyone in the organization is pursuing the same short-term objectives and long-term goals. Organizations are dysfunctional when internal stakeholders are pitted against each other in zero-sum games for personal income, budgets, space, personnel, power, etc. Providers cannot reduce costs of top-quality health services if employees and business partners are competing. On the other hand, aligned enterprises have accomplished the difficult transition from win–lose to win–win.

The organizations in the previous case studies have done a remarkable job in eliminating competition among their stakeholders. They have created teams, for example, in which physicians, nurses, and pharmacists are "working for the good of the order" because all share in the rewards of performance improvement and organizational success. Leaders should be sure that teamwork is part of the organizational culture. Most providers will discover room for improvement in this area and should be sure that their organization has the right resources, internal or external, as appropriate, for making necessary changes to establish team-work as a core value.

The medical staff is employed by the health system in most of the previously documented case studies. In employed physician situations, doctors do not have private practices that are competing with the hospital. The chief executives in most of these organizations are also physicians. An employed medical staff and physicians in top leadership positions are becoming common features of health systems recognized as the best in the country (see Chapter 5). This factor says something important about alignment as a CSF.

Finally, trustees and employed senior executives need to ensure that the payment system does not become an impediment to alignment. For example, disease management and prevention programs are valuable tools for lowering costs, but they can be difficult to implement if third-party reimbursement favors expensive episodic care. Leaders need to become actively involved in working with health plans to align payment with cost and quality objectives.

Leadership

The organizations surveyed for this book have the great fortune of strong leadership. The officials responsible for strategic direction—board members, chief management executives, medical and nursing staff officers, and physician champions—have a viable vision of the organization's potential, and they act accordingly. They know that standardizing quality and reducing costs are essential for survival and growth. (Actually, some of their organizations probably have enough resources, through big endowments and royalties, to survive for a long time without responding to the marketplace imperatives. The fact that they are responding reflects the true professionalism that should be motivating all providers to improve, even if the marketplace did not demand it.)

These leaders are also looking beyond their own organizations to the future of health care in general and the needs of their own market areas in particular. They drive their organizations to respond to the expectations of purchasers, payers, and consumers. Community benefit is a major motivation, which facilitates appropriate collaboration with other stakeholders on all sides of the marketplace.

One attribute clearly stands out as a common descriptor of successful organizations' leaders: sustained commitment. The leaders recognize that pursuit of efficiency and effectiveness is a long-term commitment, and they are willing to take personal and professional risks to push their organizations to national prominence. These executives and clinicians are relentless in their pursuit of improvements in cost and quality. Consequently, they are eager, willing, and able to move their organizations through the inevitable "rough patches" and early stages of work. Their commitment is sustained over time and across the enterprise, regardless of the roadblocks, because they know that performance improvement is the right and necessary thing to do.

Accountability

The remarkable accomplishments presented in this work's case studies were uniformly data-driven and IT-facilitated. Leaders set achievable, quantifiable goals. Then, they collected and analyzed meaningful numbers to gauge actual performance against stated, measurable objectives. Processes were continually refined until they yielded cost reductions and the desired level of quality. Then, for reasons just presented in the discussion on flexibility as a CSF, the process started over because efficiency and effectiveness are moving targets.

A quantitative definition of accountability may not, at first, come to mind, but it is paramount when the goals are efficiency and effectiveness. An organization must have numbers to judge performance. In addition, stakeholders on the demand side of the marketplace are demanding more numbers for comparing the cost and quality of competing providers. Many customers will ultimately select their providers by assessing the value of what they receive for money they spend on health care. This is the classic accountability of the law of the marketplace, as covered in basic economics courses.

Accountability is often linked to transparency in contemporary discussions of health policy. Transparency isn't listed as a CSF because it is not essential to the economic concepts of efficiency and effectiveness. A secretive (i.e., nontransparent) organization could be the least-cost producer of the top-quality good in a marketplace. As a rule, however, transparency is a concept that is wise in most circumstances. Organizations that are efficient and effective have nothing to hide and should publicize their accomplishments with great pride.

Creativity

Our case studies show that cost and quality leaders were impatient with the traditional ways of producing health care. They did not like the implications of continuing business as usual. They embraced the challenge of doing something new, different, and better. After all, obedience to tradition explains many of the problems in today's medical marketplace.

America's leaders in efficiency and effectiveness are not only eager to break the mold, but to shape a new health care system in a spirit of self-improvement and social responsibility. They are formulating visionary—even daring—responses to the imperatives of the 21st century marketplace. Creativity is a CSF. Now, on to the paradox....

| EIGHT |

RESOLVING THE PARADOX: FOUNDATIONS FOR SUCCESSFUL SYSTEM REFORM

The first chapter of this book showed how hospitals, health systems, and medical groups are entering uncharted economic territory at the beginning of the 21st century. Subsequent chapters have focused on operational changes that most providers must make to stay in business in the new and different marketplace. This final chapter identifies corresponding actions that must be taken by purchasers, payers, politicians, policy makers, and consumers if the U.S. health care system is to negotiate successfully through the turbulent times ahead. It reflects a hopeful focus on what all stakeholders can do together to make things right. Nothing is to be gained by approaches to reform that cast blame on stakeholders who have allegedly done things wrong.

Of course, providers are not unaccustomed to confronting new external challenges over time. Purchasers and payers fought "skyrocketing" costs of health care with a cascade of contradictory policies and approaches in the last 30 years of the 20th century—prepaid group health plans, regulation, and price controls in the 1970s, deregulation and competition in the 1980s, and managed care in the 1990s. Providers had to adapt to each shift in signals from the demand side of the marketplace, but they could always count on getting just enough additional revenue to cover costs of compliance with the new rules and to conceal their own inefficiencies. Health care's share of the gross domestic product increased every year, in spite of purchasers' threats that they could not or would not pay any more.

Historically, the black clouds on the horizon always had a silver lining that allowed providers to weather the storm. However, as mentioned early in this book, the silver lining is starting to disappear and will probably be gone within a few years. Fundamental changes in the economy will likely stop the flow of additional real (i.e., inflation-adjusted) dollars into health care. All but the lucky providers—those with "trust funds" or other exceptional economic advantages—need to become efficient and effective to stay in the business of health care. (Even lucky providers have an ethical and professional obligation to become efficient and effective.) Efficiency, effectiveness, and e-transformation are imperative under the circumstances.

The Paradox

Efficiency, effectiveness, and e-transformation won't happen just because they are the right things to do—or even if they're required. Leaders must make decisions and take actions that cause their organizations to move purposefully in these directions. Meeting the e-imperatives will require substantial investments in education and technology...at the very same time when surplus revenues are disappearing. The majority of providers have only enough money to meet current expenses, with no surplus to retrain staff or to install IT systems that would assure their long-run survival. Hence, the paradox: *As a precondition of staying in business by becoming efficient and effective, most providers must make investments they cannot afford.* A classic catch-22. Damned if you do, and damned if you don't. There's only one way out of the morass, and it is blocked.

Many readers have probably been wondering when this point would finally be addressed. Health care leaders wouldn't dispute the desirability of producing consistently great medical care as inexpensively as possible, but they might disagree with a decision to position this goal as a strategic imperative for their organizations. As mentioned in the Preface, some leaders said they would only be interested in this book if government required the actions prescribed. Otherwise, these leaders believe that the difficulties of becoming efficient and effective through digital transformation would be greater than any resulting rewards.

Obviously, something must be done differently to resolve the paradox. Political conservatives' solution, reducing costs and improving quality through private competition without direct government involvement, is hard to take seriously. Health care's problems are the result of cumulative market failures, as evidenced by cynical health care leaders who would only pursue efficiency and effectiveness under government orders. Ironically, significant public funds have been spent over the past decade on so-called private market reforms. These private-sector demonstration programs have not reduced costs or produced superior quality. In addition, one-half of all health care dollars now come through the government. The dynamics of privatizing this industry are simply unimaginable. John Maynard Keynes' famous observation about the long-run takes on new meaning here. We would all be dead long before a shift of this magnitude could be accomplished.

On the other hand, political liberals are equally disoriented when they advance proposals limited to pumping more government dollars into universal access to provide "inexpensive, top-quality health care for all Americans." They are proposing demand-side solutions for supply-side problems. American health care became considerably more expensive as government spending advanced from 20 percent of the total when Medicare was created in 1965 to 50 percent today. Simply proposing more government reimbursement as the solution to cost and quality problems makes about as much sense as fighting a fire with gasoline. Medicare is one of the most cost-effective health plans, but its success in restraining prices is also the #1 cause of the paradox. Government has slowed the growth of medical expenditures by exercising the power of its purse—not by well-researched programs to help providers become efficient and effective. Federal programs that have meaningfully addressed cost and quality have been woefully underfunded and politically suppressed.

Regrettably, the current debate on health care reform seems to be a battle between two unpromising and uncompromising political positions. The problems of cost and quality will not be solved any time soon if either side wins, as long as neither side has a workable plan to overcome the paradox. A fresh and feasible approach is clearly needed before progress can be made. The proposals that follow seek to move the debate in a productive direction.

Wishful Thinking: A Hill–Burton Program for the 21st Century

The United States faced a similar paradox in the mid-20th century, and government resolved it with a remarkably successful private–public partnership. World War II halted post-depression renewal of the U.S. economy, including regeneration of the health sector. The capacity of civilian hospitals was cut dramatically because so many health professionals were diverted to military service. At the same time, the scientific foundations of health care were transformed by the development of antibiotics in the 1930s and subsequent advances in surgery. Antibiotics suddenly saved the lives of millions of Americans who would have died of infectious disease, allowing them to live long enough to experience degenerative diseases (e.g., coronary and vascular conditions, cancer).

The function of a hospital changed correspondingly, from a facility that cared for people with infectious diseases until the 1930s to a facility treating people with degenerative disease after World War II. Doctors and nurses returned to civilian life ready to provide a new kind of care that hospitals were not designed to support. The start of the baby boom and urbanization also meant that the United States did not have enough hospitals to meet the demands of a rapidly growing population. Hence, the paradox of the mid-1900s—a new and different infrastructure was needed, but hospitals did not have any spare money to finance the conversion because they had no reserves after World War II.

Congress created the Hill–Burton program in 1946 for the specific purpose of building new hospitals that efficiently and effectively supported the delivery of new medical services. (The government even hired architects to prepare approved blueprints for Hill–Burton hospitals, which explains the nearly identical appearance of community hospitals built from the 1950s through the 1970s.) Hill–Burton was not a federal "give away." It required communities to match the federal funds by raising significant local capital and to follow the program's plans. The community organization was responsible for scaling its hospital to the population's projected needs.

Imagine a serious national effort to jump-start investment in IT and training that would reduce operating costs and produce consistent quality within individual organizations. The Hill–Burton program could be a model for overcoming the current paradox of health care. Good preliminary plans for the IT infrastructure of 21st century health care have already been developed collaboratively by a variety of public and private organizations. Working "blueprints" and appropriate technologies for digital transformation are available, but nothing has been done to guarantee the financing. The idea of community-based efforts to match federal dollars with local funds to implement specific plans is an idea whose time ought to have come.

Regional health information organizations (RHIO) would be explicitly excluded from a Hill–Burton type approach to digital transformation. Providers must become efficient and effective internally before geographic marketplaces might reap any benefits from data sharing. Regional information exchange won't solve any problems if the participating providers are inefficient and ineffective. The business and clinical cases for RHIOs can be revisited after providers have mastered costs and quality—if information sharing isn't already being adequately managed by the likes of Google and Microsoft.

The problem with this vision is the near-zero probability of finding new federal money, for reasons explained in Chapter 1. The only realistic possibility would be redirecting funds to health care from existing uses. The federal government currently spends more than enough money on some activities that ought to be discontinued. The United States needs political leaders who would reallocate some authorized funds to an IT program modeled on Hill–Burton. Although this policy recommendation is based on wishful thinking, it is certainly a thought worth considering.

Foundations for Policy and Progress

This book's fundamental financial forecast—the impending end of real growth in providers' overall incomes—could end up being the good news. Hospitals and medical groups would be slitting their own throats if purchasers and payers ultimately force providers to pass on the savings from becoming efficient and effective. The demand side of the marketplace could kill health care by reducing expenditures simply for the sake of reducing expenditures. Widespread closure of hospitals and medical groups would occur if private and public payers were to cut reimbursement below the break-even point for the industry.

Third-party payers have reasonably defended previous payment reductions by arguing that they should not subsidize health care's high costs and low quality. They argued that providers could ignore efficiency and effectiveness because payments were effectively made with a "blank check." The federal government explicitly replaced retrospective cost-based reimbursement with prospective reimbursement in 1983 because it wanted to force hospitals to live within fixed budgets. The same policy was extended to physician payments six years later. Payers and policy makers have correctly asserted that the supply side was wasting money, and their subsequent tightening of reimbursement could be seen as punishment for the waste. They have assumed providers would respond rationally by learning how to produce uniform, top-quality health care for less money. This assumption has been wrong for the past 25 years.

Reimbursement policy has never been specifically designed to push providers toward clear and objective performance goals. Reformers have simplistically assumed that providers would be forced into clinical and economic shape if put on a restricted monetary diet. In the absence of coordinated incentives and empowerment to change their organizational behaviors, most providers have continued to operate with abundant waste. The situation reminds us of equally simplistic efforts to reduce the average American's abundant waistline with low-fat or nonfat foods. The more "lite" food people eat, the heavier they become, if they do not make appropriate behavioral changes. For the same reason, reimbursement reform needs to include specific incentives that promote desired change in the way providers behave as organizations. Reimbursement reform should be linked to behavior change.

No stakeholder on either side of the market has ever determined what health care would cost if it were produced efficiently and effectively. Policy makers don't have the slightest idea how much money would be needed to support a rational health system. Most just assume it would be less than what is currently being spent. This assumption might be wrong. For example, public health and preventive medicine are woefully underfunded in the United States. If the costs of much-needed "wellness care" exceeded the money wasted on "sickness care," then a rational health system would need more resources than the current (i.e., irrational) system.

The 17 Percent Solution

Nobody knows whether 17 percent of GDP is an appropriate amount to spend on health care. The economy can, however, afford 17 percent. (Health care falls far down on the list of reasons for the current disarray in the U.S. economy. Expenditures on health care have reached the limit of what Americans are willing to pay, but the shaky economy has resulted from other forces—most notably, U.S. addiction to foreign oil, a growing trade deficit, massive public and private debt, and dysfunctional investment markets.) Unfortunately, many Americans do not get health care they need; many get health care they do not need; and quite a few get bad health care, whether they need it or not.

The implied need for a study to determine optimal allocation of resources to health care will be appealing to consulting firms and think tanks, but the United States does not have the luxury of time to do this research. Conducting a comprehensive study would require several years; hospitals and physicians cannot wait that long to begin solving their problems. Further, the clinical dynamics of health care will have changed so much in the interim that the study's results would be irrelevant by the time they could be reported. A research initiative is not a solution. Getting hospitals to use *existing* tools of performance improvement is a solution.

Whether 17 percent is an appropriate or inappropriate amount for our nation to spend on health care, the dollar amount of spending it represents currently provides just enough money to keep providers in business as usual. Hospitals and medical groups need to make major investments in IT in order to do their business better, that is, to solve the problems of cost and quality. Finally, providers will not likely be able to finance these investments with incremental revenues from growth because the medical economy will not be growing. Since a Hill–Burton proposal is wishful thinking, macroeconomic analysis suggests the essential investments in process change and information infrastructure must be made with part of the existing 17 percent. Trying to cut below 17 percent without first resolving the cost and quality issues would not be progress. The real challenge is to see how much more value can be produced with 17 percent of the GDP committed to health care. For that respectable sum, the United States could build the best health care system in the world—if done efficiently, effectively, and electronically.

Policy Prescription #1: Preserve Providers' Revenue

Most providers will struggle to reallocate resources within their organization's piece of the fixed GDP pie. Threats of a smaller piece would prove devastating because e-transformation must be financed with money saved by improvements in efficiency and effectiveness. Therefore, providers must be able to count on stable income in exchange for undertaking the difficult tasks of process improvement and clinical transformation. Purchasers, payers, and patients must recognize and respect this catch-22. They must consequently stabilize real reimbursement for hospitals and medical groups that are making necessary changes to produce efficient and effective health care. (Stabilization will need to be adjusted for relative changes in volume over time, e.g., if a hospital gains market share, its share of real income in the marketplace should rise proportionally.) The growing practice of across-the-board cuts in reimbursement will only torpedo progressive providers' efforts to become efficient and effective.

Consequently, policy makers and health care industry leaders need to define the criteria that will justify constant real (i.e., uncut) reimbursement to provider organizations that are doing all the right things. Some observers will argue that performance-based reimbursement will accomplish this goal, but it will not. Pay for performance gives only a modest premium to providers that meet a relatively small number of performance goals. What's more, P4P does not represent a global commitment to maintain real incomes for providers that are transforming everything about their operations. In other words, while the concept of P4P represents an opening to new thinking around reimbursement, P4P as it now exists will not take us where we need to go as a system. Instead, the new compact around reimbursement should be something akin to the special status given to critical access hospitals (CAH) in rural areas, disproportionate share hospitals (DSH), or providers in high-wage areas.

Assurance of reimbursement stability should require providers to implement programs for performance improvement and clinical transformation and to invest in IT systems that support these activities. A federally funded special commission of government agencies and respected nongovernmental organizations with developed expertise in efficiency, effectiveness, and e-transformation should be established to develop eligibility criteria. The commission would not need to invent anything; it would be an aggregator of existing tools that have been proven to reduce costs and ensure specified quality (e.g., management techniques used by programs identified in the previous chapters). The commission's report would define quantifiable criteria for certifying providers engaged in enterprise-wide transformation.

To launch movement in the right direction, the reimbursement stabilization effort could be named the Cost and Quality Performance program (CQP, just as DSH designates the Disproportionate Share Hospitals program). Compliant providers would receive CQP designation upon proving they have implemented and are using consensus-approved tools and technologies for performance improvement across the enterprise. Much work needs to be done to turn this concept into a functioning program. Another book could be written on this recommendation alone. However, the authors' respective roles as medical economist and journalist demonstrate how to merge theory and practice into a feasible proposal for solving a serious problem. Purchasers, payers, and providers should start working together right away to turn the CQP into a working solution.

Building a foundation for efficiency and effectiveness should be a nonpartisan goal. If politics threatens to get in the way, the commission for closing military bases could be used as a model to make sure that the job gets done for the right reasons. The criteria for CQP designation could be developed in a year. Hospitals and medical groups need assurance as soon as possible that they can retain and reallocate the internal savings they produce by becoming efficient and effective. They will have no economic incentive to make the required investments in improvement if their reward is lower reimbursement. Conversely, most providers need assurances of stability before making the dramatic changes to become efficient and effective. A properly crafted Cost and Quality Performance program would provide the assurance that most hospitals need to see past the paradox and respond to the imperatives.

Policy Prescription #2: Create Efficiency in Payment Processes

Inefficiency is not restricted to providers on the supply side of the medical marketplace. A lot of economic waste is generated on the demand side by business practices of purchasers and payers. For example, third-party organizations cause considerable sums to be spent unproductively on personnel to process claims. The Health Insurance Portability and Accountability Act of 1996 (HIPAA) may create the impression of industry-wide efficiency because it imposes electronic claims processing, but thousands of clerks move tons of paper just beneath the digital surface on both sides of the marketplace.

Hospitals and medical groups are absolutely correct in stating that many of their inefficiencies are forced upon them by the reimbursement system. They waste a lot of money meeting the requirements of an antiquated system for paying providers' bills. The current approach to processing health care claims is a classic Rube Goldberg system, engineered to accomplish a relatively simple task in a highly complex way. It definitely contributes to the high price of health care in the United States.

Hence, isolating and reallocating the waste in the health care system requires major redesign of the payment process. Providers cannot single-handedly accomplish the tasks of reforming health care because some significant operational problems are rooted in the policies and procedures for reimbursement. Hospitals and medical groups can reasonably ask the payer community to begin modernizing reimbursement as a perfectly appropriate quid pro quo for demonstrable progress in producing consistently good health care as inexpensively as possible.

Conclusion: Challenge for Collaboration

Examining issues around paradox and imperatives for payers lies beyond the scope of this book, which has been purposefully provider-focused. Nevertheless, leaders from government and private health plans will hopefully respond to this book with the same spirit of self-improvement expected from providers. Further, hospitals and medical groups will expect payers to change reimbursement procedures that create waste for providers. Finally, eliminating waste from the payment process is necessary for building the best health care system that 17 percent of GDP can buy.

Of course, providers face the biggest challenges and have the most work to do. Their processes for producing health care must be transformed before any other approaches to reform can be successful. Extending access to all Americans won't produce a better health care system if providers and payers are wasting resources. If all health care's stakeholders would look forward to what they can accomplish *working together* toward the common goal of ensuring efficient and effective health care—rather than looking backward to cast blame for a failing system—the United States really could build the best health care system in the world.

Suggested Reading

Robert Barry, PhD., Amy C. Murcko, APRN, and Clifford E. Brubaker, PhD. *The Six Sigma Book for Healthcare: Improving Outcomes by Reducing Errors.* Chicago: Health Administration Press, 2002.

Jeffrey K. Liker, PhD. *The Toyota Way: 14 Management Principles from the Worlds Greatest Manufacturer.* New York: McGraw-Hill, 2003.

Jeffrey K. Liker, PhD, ed. *Becoming Lean: Inside Stories of U.S. Manufacturers.* New York: Productivity Press, 1997.

Jeffrey Morgan. *Creating Lean Corporations: Reengineering from the Bottom Up to Eliminate Waste.* New York: Productivity Press, 2005.

Edward J. O'Connor, PhD. and C. Marlena Fiol, PhD. *Reclaiming Your Future: Entrepreneurial Thinking in Health Care.* Tampa, FL: American College of Physician Executives, 2002.

Mark A. Nash, Sheila R. Poling, Sophronia Ward. *Using Lean for Faster Six Sigma Results: A Synchronized Approach.* New York: Productivity Press, 2006.

Patrice L. Spath. *Leading Your Healthcare Organization to Excellence: A Guide to Using the Baldrige Criteria.* Chicago: Health Administration Press, 2004.

James P. Womack and Daniel T. Jones. *Lean Thinking: Banish Waste and Create Wealth in Your Corporation.* New York: Simon & Schuster, 2003.

Index

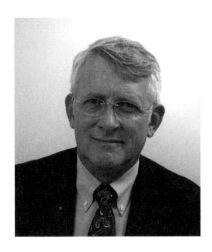

Jeffrey C. Bauer, PhD, is a Chicago-based partner in health care management consulting and director of the health care futures practice for Affiliated Computer Services, Inc. (ACS). As a consultant with more than 15 years of experience, he assists hospitals and other provider organizations with strategic planning and visioning, leadership education, technology assessment, and service line transformation. Dr. Bauer also spent 17 years as a professor at two medical schools and served as Health Policy Adviser to the governor of Colorado. A nationally respected medical economist and health futurist, Dr. Bauer has published 150 articles, books, and videos. He speaks frequently to national audiences about key trends in health care, medical science, technology, reimbursement, information systems, public policy, health reform, and creative problem solving. In his numerous publications and presentations, he forecasts the future of health care and describes practical, creative approaches to improving the delivery system. Dr. Bauer is quoted often in the national press and writes regularly for professional journals that cover the business of health care. He was a Ford Foundation Independent Scholar, a Fulbright Scholar (Switzerland), and a Kellogg Foundation National Fellow. He holds a BA from Colorado College and a PhD in economics from the University of Colorado at Boulder.

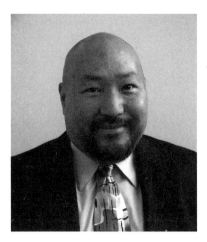

Mark Hagland is a national award-winning health care journalist with nearly 20 years' experience covering a diverse array of industry issues, from health care policy to provider-payer relations to quality, strategic planning, managed care, and information technology topics. A former Executive Editor of *Hospitals & Health Networks* magazine, he has been an independent health care journalist since 1996. In 1997, he was the national winner in the trade publication category of the National Institute for Health Care Management's Fourth Annual Health Care Journalism Award, for a cover story he wrote for *California Medicine* on the challenges of the IPA model of physician governance. His three-part cover story series on patient safety issues for *Healthcare Informatics* received a bronze regional award from the American Society of Business Publication Editors in 2006. And the article he and Jeffrey Bauer co-wrote for *Healthcare Financial Management* on the emergence of consumer-directed health care won the Helen Yeger/L. Vann Seawell Best Article Award for 2006/2007 from the Healthcare Financial Management Association. Hagland continues to write for a wide variety of professional publications in health care and to speak to a range of executive and governance audiences. He has a BA in English from the University of Wisconsin and a master's degree in journalism from the Medill School of Journalism at Northwestern University. He lives in Chicago.